The Vagus Nerve

The Ultimate Guide to Understanding and Stimulating the Vagus Nerve to Improve Well-being, Mental Clarity, and Emotional Resilience

Written by *Adrienne Fox*

Author: Chair Yoga For Seniors

THE VAGUS NERVE COMMUNITY - STAYHEALTHY

Explore the vagus nerve, a crucial aspect of achieving harmony and balance in your body. "Vital Vagus" is a journey into understanding one of your body's most influential nerves. With a blend of scientific insights and practical advice, this guide is tailored for those who face the challenges of modern stress, anxiety, and overall health concerns. Whether you're a busy professional struggling with stress or a parent seeking emotional stability, this book offers a path to not only understanding but also mastering your body's innate healing powers.

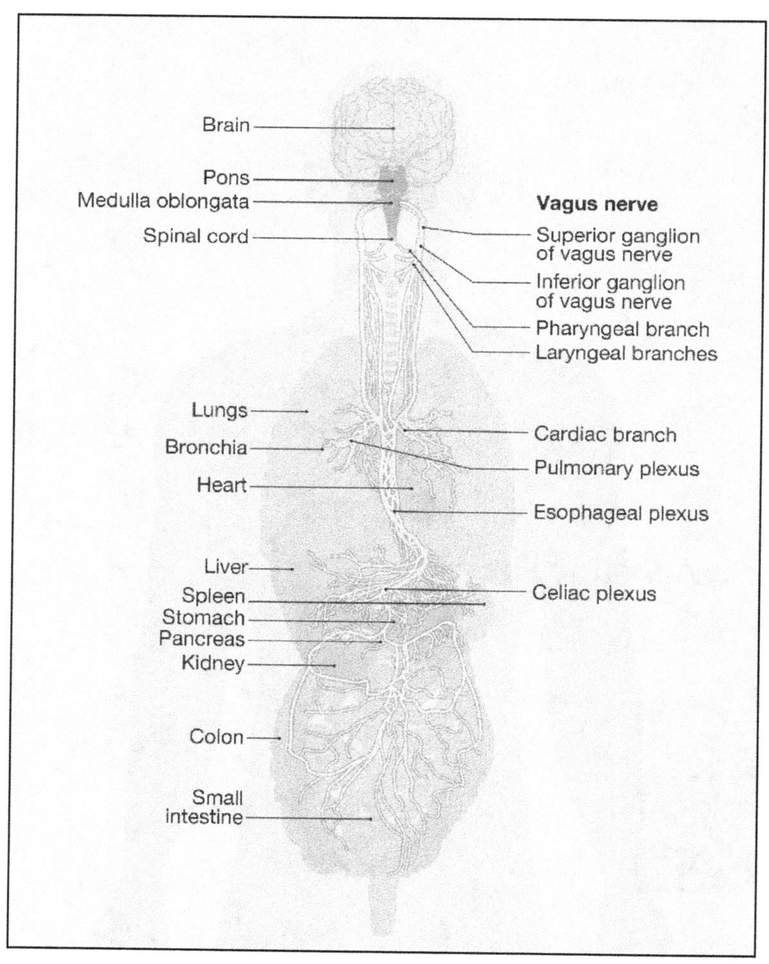

Table of Contents

Chapter 1: Introduction to the Vagus Nerve

1.1 Understanding the Vagus Nerve: Function and Importance

1.1.1: The Anatomy of the Vagus Nerve

The vagus nerve, identified as cranial nerve X, is an integral part of the autonomic nervous system.

It is the longest cranial nerve in the human body, stretching from the brainstem through the neck and into the abdomen. This nerve plays a primary role in connecting the brain to major organs, including the heart, lungs, and digestive tract.

It consists of both sensory (afferent) and motor (efferent) fibers, making it a mixed nerve that not only transmits signals to the organs but also conveys sensory information back to the brain. Its extensive reach and complex structure allow it to regulate a vast array of bodily functions, underscoring its importance in maintaining overall physiological balance.

1.1.2: Key Functions of the Vagus Nerve

The vagus nerve is crucial in controlling the body's parasympathetic response, which is also known as the 'rest and digest' system.

It is essential for managing heart rate, controlling muscle movements in the gastrointestinal tract, and controlling respiratory rate.

This nerve's influence on the heart is particularly significant, as it helps to lower the heart rate and reduce the intensity of cardiac contractions, thereby exerting a calming effect on the body.

In the digestive system, it stimulates muscles to contract and relax, aiding in the process of digestion and promoting efficient nutrient absorption and waste elimination. Additionally, the vagus nerve is involved in mood regulation and stress response, further highlighting its multifaceted role in maintaining physiological and psychological equilibrium.

1.1.3: The Vagus Nerve and Mind-Body Connection

The intricate mind-body connection depends heavily on the vagus nerve. It operates as a fast communication between the brain and the gastrointestinal system, an interaction often termed the gut-brain axis.

This connection has significant implications for mental health, as the state of the gut can directly influence mood and emotional well-being. The nerve's sensory capabilities enable it to relay information about the body's internal state to the brain, impacting emotional responses and stress levels. Understanding this connection opens new paths for treating various mental health disorders, stressing the significance of holistic approaches that reflect both mental and physical health.

Section 1.1.4: The Science Behind Vagal Tone

The activity of the vagus nerve is called vagal tone and is commonly assessed by Heart Rate Variability (HRV), which is the difference in time between each heartbeat. A higher vagal tone is associated with a body's better ability to relax after stress and is often linked to positive emotions and good physical health. Conversely, low vagal tone can be indicative of various health issues, including cardiovascular conditions and increased susceptibility to stress and mood disorders. Research in this area highlights the potential of interventions aimed at increasing vagal tone, such as breathing exercises and meditation, as effective tools for enhancing overall health and resilience.

1.2 How Vagus Nerve Health Impacts Your Life

1.2.1: Recognizing an Imbalanced Vagus Nerve

Various physical and psychological symptoms can be caused by a vague nerve that is unbalanced or dysfunctional. Physiologically, it may lead to digestive issues such as irritable Bowel Syndrome (IBS), heartburn, or slow gastric emptying, given its crucial role in controlling the digestive tract muscles. On the cardiovascular front, vagal imbalance can result in an irregular heartbeat or heart rate variability, potentially elevating the risk of heart-related conditions. From a mental health perspective, the vagus nerve's dysfunction can contribute to heightened stress levels, anxiety, and mood swings. The reason for this is its significant impact on the parasympathetic nervous system, which adjusts the body's relaxation responses. Individuals with a poorly functioning vagus nerve might find it difficult to cope with stress, recover from stressful events, or manage their emotional responses effectively. Acknowledging these signs is vital for timely intervention and management.

1.2.2: Vagus Nerve and Overall Health

The health of the vagus nerve is intrinsically linked to overall well-being. A well-functioning vagus nerve supports the body's "rest and digest" functions, facilitating efficient digestion, steady heart rate, and relaxed breathing patterns. Plays a vital role in regulating inflammation, a factor behind many chronic diseases. Reduced inflammatory response through proper vagal function can reduce the risk of conditions such as arthritis, heart disease, and possibly some autoimmune disorders. Moreover, the vagus nerve's influence on the gut-brain axis means it has a substantial impact on mental health. Optimal vagal tone can enhance mood regulation and resilience against stress-related disorders, emphasizing the nerve's holistic contribution to health.

1.2.3: Psychological and Emotional Aspects

The vagus nerve's impact extends beyond physical health, deeply affecting psychological and emotional well-being. Its role in the parasympathetic nervous system means it's directly involved in managing stress responses. High vagal tone is often associated with greater emotional regulation, calmness, and an ability to maintain a balanced mood. Conversely, low vagal activity can contribute to heightened stress, anxiety, and susceptibility to mood disorders.

Understanding the vagus nerve's role in emotional health is essential for creating effective methods to manage stress, anxiety, and depression. This knowledge has led to innovative treatments like Vagus Nerve Stimulation (VNS), which has shown promise in treating various psychological disorders.

1.2.4: Vagus Nerve in Daily Life

The state of the vagus nerve can be influenced by daily habits and lifestyle choices. Poor dietary habits, chronic stress, lack of physical activity, and inadequate sleep can negatively impact vagal tone. Conversely, practices such as regular exercise, mindful eating, stress management techniques, and adequate rest can enhance vagal function. Straightforward activities like deep breathing exercises, yoga, and meditation have been proven to stimulate the vagus nerve, advocating relaxation and reducing stress. Moreover, maintaining social connections and engaging in laughter and positive interactions can also improve vagal tone, underscoring the importance of a holistic approach to vagus nerve health. By integrating these practices into daily life, anyone can proactively support their vagus nerve health, contributing to improved overall well-being.

In essence, the health of the vagus nerve is pivotal in maintaining a balance between physical and emotional well-being. Its role extends from the direct regulation of bodily functions to influencing our capacity to manage stress and emotional states. Recognizing the signs of vagal imbalance and incorporating lifestyle practices that support its function can lead to significant improvements in overall health and quality of life.

Chapter 2: The Vagus Nerve and Stress

2.1: The Science of Stress and the Vagus Nerve

2.1.1: Understanding Stress Response

A cascade of physiological responses is a result of stress, which is a common element of modern life. When faced with stress, the body's immediate reaction is the activation of the sympathetic nervous system, often termed the "fight or flight" response. This response is designed to prepare the body for perceived threats by raising heart rate, redirecting blood flow to crucial muscles, and releasing stress hormones like cortisol and adrenaline. However, this response, while vital in acute situations, can become detrimental when persistently activated, leading to chronic stress. Here, we delve into the intricacies of how the body responds to stress, laying the foundation for understanding the vital counterbalancing role of the vagus nerve.

2.1.2: Vagus Nerve - The Body's Natural Stress Buffer

As the primary component of the parasympathetic nervous system, the vagus nerve acts as a natural counterweight to the stress response. It acts as a brake to the sympathetic system, promoting the "rest and digest" functions. This section explores how the vagus nerve helps in reducing heart rate, lowering blood pressure, and calming the body after stress exposure. The concept of the 'vagal brake' is pivotal, as it illustrates how the nerve can rapidly swing the body from a state of heightened stress to one of calm and relaxation. This ability of the vagus nerve to modulate stress responses is crucial for maintaining physiological and emotional balance.

2.1.3: The Role of Vagal Tone in Stress Resilience

Vagal tone, a measure of the vagus nerve's activity, is directly linked to how effectively the body can manage and recover from stress.

High vagal tone is associated with greater variability in heart rate, which is indicative of a healthy and resilient cardiovascular system, able to quickly adapt to varying stress levels. Studies examined show that individuals with higher vagal tone generally have better emotional regulation capabilities and are less susceptible to the negative impacts of stress. The ability to maintain a high vagal tone is thus seen as a key factor in building resilience against the physiological and psychological effects of stress.

2.1.4: Stress-Induced Vagal Dysfunction

Chronic stress can have a deep impact on the vagus nerve's functioning, leading to what is often referred to as 'vagus nerve fatigue.' This condition is characterized by a diminished ability of the vagus nerve to effectively regulate the body's stress response. Symptoms may include digestive disorders, heart rhythm irregularities, and an inability to relax or recover from stress. This section explores the consequences of prolonged stress on vagal health, the potential for developing chronic conditions, and how recognizing and addressing these early signs of vagal dysfunction can be crucial for long-term health and well-being.

2.1.5: Polyvagal Theory

Polyvagal Theory provides a deeper understanding of the human body's response systems through the lens of the vagus nerve, emphasizing the importance of autonomic nervous system functioning in shaping our experiences of safety and threat. Here's a more detailed look into the three developmental stages of response proposed by Dr. Stephen Porges:

1. ***Immobilization (Dorsal Vagus Complex)***: This oldest response involves the dorsal vagus nerve, which activates during extreme stress or danger, leading to a "freeze" state where the body may shut down or dissociate. This response is primal and used as a last resort when the body perceives life-threatening situations.

2. ***Mobilization (Sympathetic Nervous System)***: When a threat is detected and more action is needed, the sympathetic nervous system kicks in, enabling the "fight or flight" response. This involves physical mobilization, such as running from danger or confronting it, facilitated by increased heart rate, blood flow, and adrenaline.

3. ***Social Engagement (Ventral Vagus Complex)***: Representing the most advanced evolutionary mechanism, this stage involves the ventral side of the vagus nerve, which is active when we perceive environments as safe. It supports social interaction and calm states, enabling us to engage with others, communicate effectively, and build social bonds.

Each of these stages reflects different evolutionary adaptations to stress and safety, highlighting the complexity of our physiological responses in various environments. This hierarchy of responses allows for a fluid, adaptable interaction with our environment, impacting emotional regulation, social behavior, and overall health.

2.2.1: Physical Symptoms of Vagal Imbalance

Recognizing physical symptoms of vagal imbalance is very important for early intervention. The vagus nerve, pivotal in regulating many bodily functions, can manifest imbalance through various signs. Common symptoms include digestive disturbances like unexplained nausea, tinnitus, bloating, and constipation, reflecting its influence on gut motility. Additionally, since the vagus nerve plays a role in heart rate regulation, symptoms can include palpitations or abnormally slow heart rate. Chronic fatigue and a sense of physical lethargy, despite adequate rest, can also indicate reduced vagal tone. Respiratory irregularities, like shallow breathing or shortness of breath without exertion, can be further signs of vagal nerve dysfunction. Understanding these symptoms is key in assessing the health of the vagus nerve and determining the need for further medical evaluation.

About Tinnitus

The relationship between tinnitus and the vagus nerve is complex, as the vagus nerve plays a critical role in modulating the body's response to stress and sensory perception, including hearing. Tinnitus is often associated with hyperactivity in certain auditory pathways in the brain, and the vagus nerve—which runs from the brainstem to many organs in the body, including the ears—can influence these auditory processes through its regulatory functions.

Here are a few ways this relationship manifests:

1. Stress and Anxiety Modulation: The vagus nerve helps regulate the parasympathetic nervous system, which is involved in the body's relaxation response. Chronic tinnitus is often worsened by stress and anxiety, which activate the sympathetic nervous system. The vagus nerve, when functioning well, promotes relaxation, potentially reducing

stress-related exacerbations of tinnitus. Vagus nerve stimulation (VNS) has been explored as a therapy to reduce the perceived volume or persistence of tinnitus through this calming effect.

2. Neuroplasticity and Auditory Perception: Studies suggest that vagus nerve stimulation may enhance neuroplasticity, which is the brain's ability to reorganize and form new neural connections. In tinnitus therapy, VNS combined with sound therapy has shown promise in helping the brain "unlearn" the abnormal sound perception that causes tinnitus, potentially reducing or alleviating symptoms over time. The idea is that stimulating the vagus nerve may help retrain the auditory cortex to ignore the tinnitus signal.

3. Modulation of Auditory Pathways: The vagus nerve interacts with several brain areas involved in auditory processing, including the auditory cortex and the limbic system (which deals with emotions). This interaction means the vagus nerve can influence how sound is processed and how the brain responds to tinnitus. By affecting these pathways, vagus nerve stimulation might help regulate the brain's response to tinnitus and reduce its perceived intensity.

2.2.2: Psychological Manifestations

The vagus nerve imbalance can significantly impact mental health. Individuals might experience heightened stress, anxiety, and mood swings. This is due to the vagus nerve's behavior in the parasympathetic nervous system and its influence on stress responses. Chronic stress or anxiety, often with no apparent external cause, can be a telltale sign of vagal dysfunction. Other psychological manifestations include difficulty in emotional regulation, feelings of being overwhelmed, and a general sense of unease or unrest. Persistent symptoms might contribute to the development of mood disorders like depression. This book aims to shed light on these psychological aspects, providing insights into how vagal health is intrinsically linked to emotional and mental well-being.

2.2.3: The Interplay Between Physical and Psychological Symptoms

The relationship between physical and psychological symptoms in vagal nerve health is complex and bidirectional. Often, physical symptoms like gut health issues can make worse mental health problems, and vice versa. Chronic stress can lead to physical manifestations of vagal imbalance, which then further feeds into the cycle of stress and anxiety, creating a feedback loop. The interconnection of these symptoms is further explored in later chapters, with the use of case studies to illustrate how they often coexist and have an impact on each other. Understanding this interplay is crucial in developing a holistic approach to addressing vagal nerve imbalance.

2.2.4: Self-Assessment Tools for Vagal Health

Empowering readers with self-assessment tools to gauge their vagal health is an essential step in self-care. There are simple and non-invasive methods to self-assess vagal tone, including observing heart rate variability and response to stress, through questionnaires. Questionnaires focusing on the frequency and severity of physical and psychological symptoms can help individuals determine their vagal health status. However, these tools are not substitutes for professional medical evaluation but rather a first step in recognizing potential issues. Encouraging people to seek professional advice for a comprehensive assessment is a key message here.

Is it possible to measure my tone from the comfort of my own home??

Tracking heart rate and breathing rate simultaneously is how vagal tone is measured.

Inhaling produces a slight increase in heart rate while exhaling produces a slight decrease. Our vagal tone is higher when there is a greater difference between our inhalation and exhalation heart rates.

How do you monitor vagal tone?

Vagal tone measurements can be performed by invasive or non-invasive procedures. Invasive procedures are rare and involve stimulating the vagus nerve through manual, respiratory, or electrical means.

Are there exercises to increase my vagal tone?

Singing, humming and gargling contests activate the vocal cord muscles and can stimulate the vagus nerve, which are interconnected and located in the back of the throat.

3.1: Managing Work Stress through Vagal Tone Improvement

3.1.1: Understanding Work-Related Stress and Vagal Tone

In today's fast-paced career world, work-related stress is a common challenge. Chronic stress not only impairs cognitive function and productivity but also negatively impacts vagal tone, affecting overall health. It's important to understand biological mechanisms of stress, particularly focusing on how the vagus nerve, as part of the parasympathetic nervous system, can mitigate stress responses. It highlights the interplay between work-induced stress and vagal tone, emphasizing the importance of maintaining a healthy vagus nerve function for professionals. The goal is to provide a foundational understanding that underscores why nurturing the vagus nerve is essential for managing work stress effectively.

3.1.2: Practical Exercises for the Workplace

Given the constraints of a professional setting, it is suggest series of practical exercises are designed to stimulate the vagus nerve without needing to step away from the desk. These include simple yet effective techniques like controlled breathing exercises, which can be done even during a busy day. They cover methods such as diaphragmatic breathing, brief guided meditation practices, and subtle neck stretches to relieve tension. The exercises are tailored to be discreet and efficient, ensuring they are feasible for implementation in any workplace environment.

(Chair Yoga Exercises on pages 18 – 19)

3.1.3: Incorporating Vagal Health into Your Work Routine

To make vagal tone improvement a sustainable part of a professional's daily routine, it is appropriate to provide strategies for integrating vagus nerve-stimulating activities into regular work habits. It's important to take short, regular breaks to practice vagal exercises, mindful eating during lunch breaks, and maintaining physical postures that support vagal health. Tips on creating routines, such as starting the day with a vagal tone-boosting activity or incorporating mini relaxation sessions between meetings, are shared to help professionals make these practices an integral part of their work life.

3.1.4: Technology and Vagal Tone

With the help of technology, one can better manage work stress by using digital tools to improve vagal tone. There are now several mobile apps and smart watches designed for stress management using meditation, breathing exercises, stretching and yoga exercises, as well as monitoring vital parameters such as heart rate variability, or night sleep and afternoon nap data.

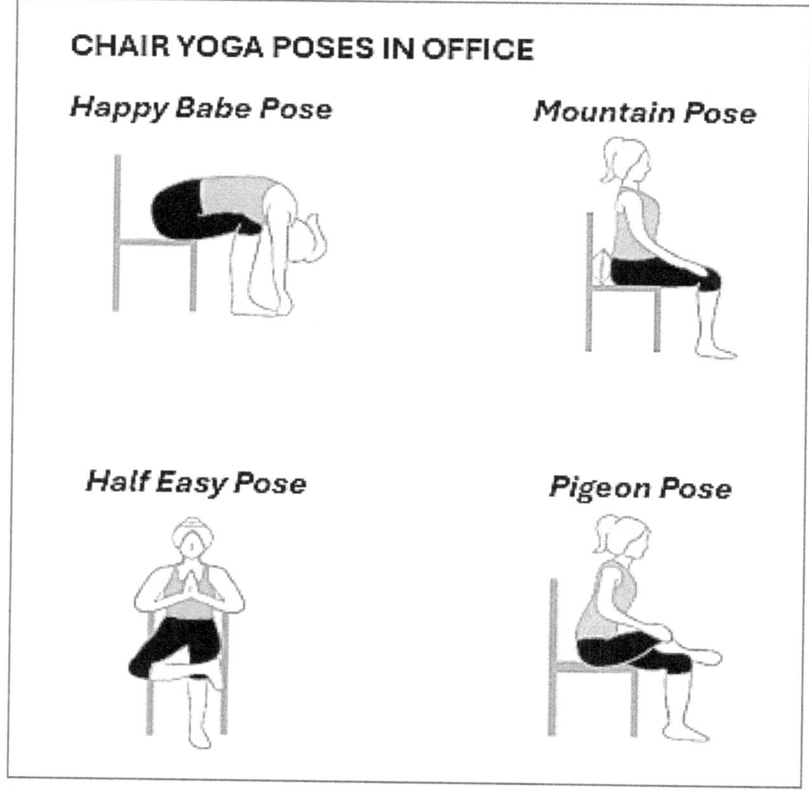

(Source Adrienne Fox Chair Yoga For Seniors)

Chair Yoga Poses in Office

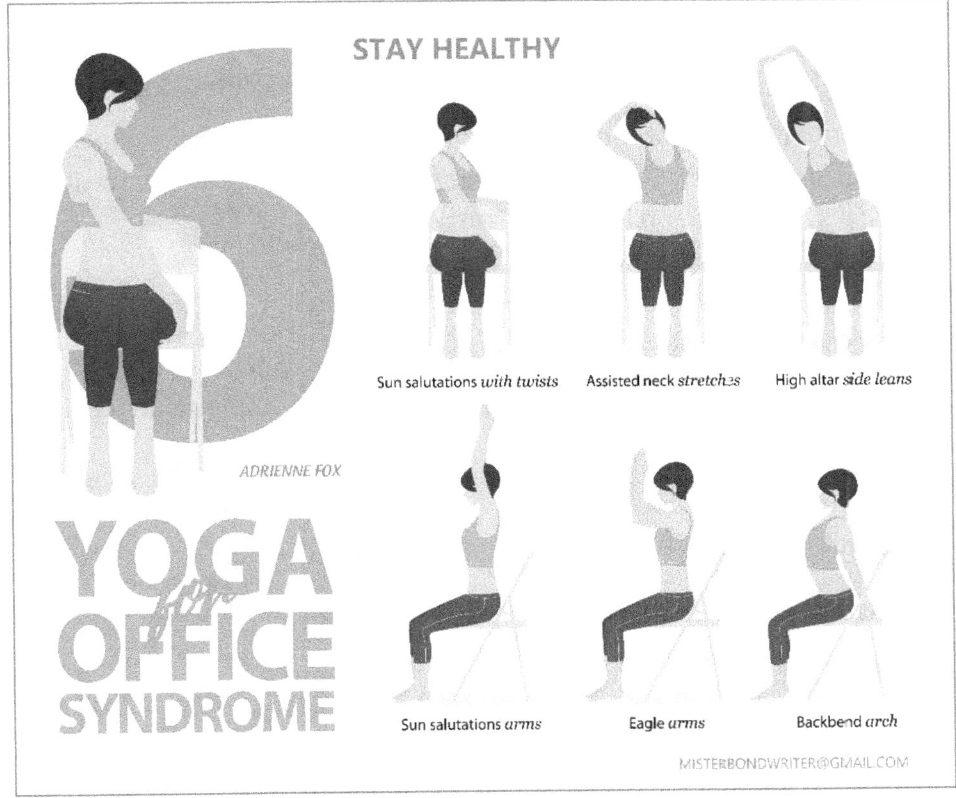

(Source StayHealthy Facebook Page)

About "Box Breathing": How to do it, benefits, and tips.

Box breathing is a profound breathing technique that can relieve stress. It's also known as "Square breathing" and is beneficial for reducing physical symptoms and improving mental focus.

1. <u>What is Box Breathing</u>?

  - It's a basic relaxation technique to return breathing to its ordinary rhythm after stress.

  - Involves four steps: breathing in, holding the breath, breathing out, and holding the breath again, always for 4 seconds.

2. <u>Benefits of Box Breathing</u>:

  - Reduces physical stress symptoms.

  - Positively influences emotions and mental well-being.

  - Increases mental clarity, energy, and focus.

  - Improves future reactions to stress.

3. <u>How to Practice Box Breathing</u>:

  - Sit comfortably with back supported and feet on the floor.

  - Close eyes, inhale in through the nose for 4 seconds, hold for 4 seconds, exhale for 4 seconds, and wait four seconds before repeating.

  - Ideally, repeat for 4 minutes or until calm.

4. <u>Additional Insights</u>:

  - Used by people in high-stress jobs like soldiers and police officers.

- Can be trained anywhere, easy to learn, and highly successful in stressful situations.

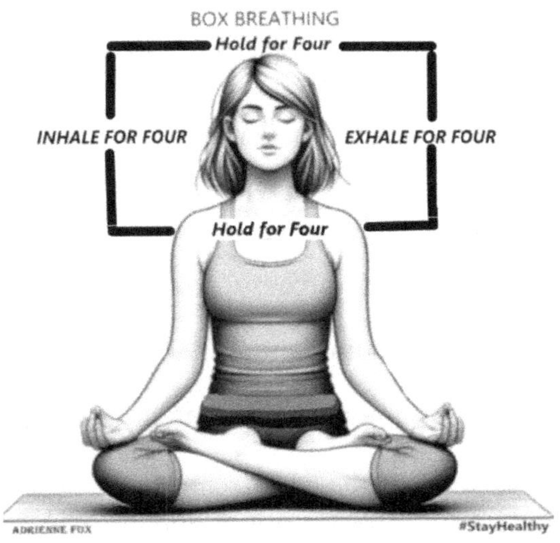

About *"BEE BREATH"*

Bee Breath, also known as **Bhramari Pranayama**, is a calming breathing technique in yoga and pranayama practices. The name "Bhramari" comes from the Sanskrit word "Bhramar," meaning "bee." In this practice, the sound made while exhaling resembles the humming of a bee, which helps create a soothing and meditative experience.

1. <u>How to Practice Bee Breath</u>:

1. Find a Comfortable Position: Sit in a quiet place, cross-legged, with your spine straight. Close your eyes and relax your shoulders.

2. Close Your Ears and Eyes: Use your thumbs to gently press the cartilage of your ears to block out external noise. You can lightly place your index fingers over your closed eyelids.

3. Inhale Deeply: Breathe in slowly and deeply through your nose.

4. Exhale with a "Hum": As you exhale, make a gentle humming sound (like a bee buzzing), keeping your mouth closed. Feel the vibrations in your head.

5. Focus on the Sound: Let your mind focus entirely on the humming sound and the vibrations it produces. This helps in calming the mind and relieving stress.

2. <u>Benefits of Bee Breath:</u>

- Calms the mind: Helps reduce anxiety, stress, and tension.

- Improves focus: Clears the mind and enhances concentration.

- Relieves anger: The calming vibrations help in soothing frustration or irritability.

- Balances emotions: Promotes emotional balance and a feeling of inner peace.

- Improves sleep: Regular practice may help with insomnia by relaxing the nervous system.

3.2: Reducing Work-Related Stress

3.2.1: Time Management and Stress Reduction

In the high-stress environment of modern professional life, effective time management is more than a skill-it is a necessity for health and well-being. It's necessary to focus on strategies for efficiently managing time and activities to minimize stress. There is a need to prioritize, of delegation and the art of saying "No" to excessive workload. There are techniques such as the Eisenhower Box (urgent- important matrix) and Pomodoro Technique that serve to optimize productivity while maintaining balance, as well as scheduling breaks and downtime to prevent burnout.

Eisenhower Matrix
Urgent-Important Matrix

<u>POMODORO TECNIQUE</u>

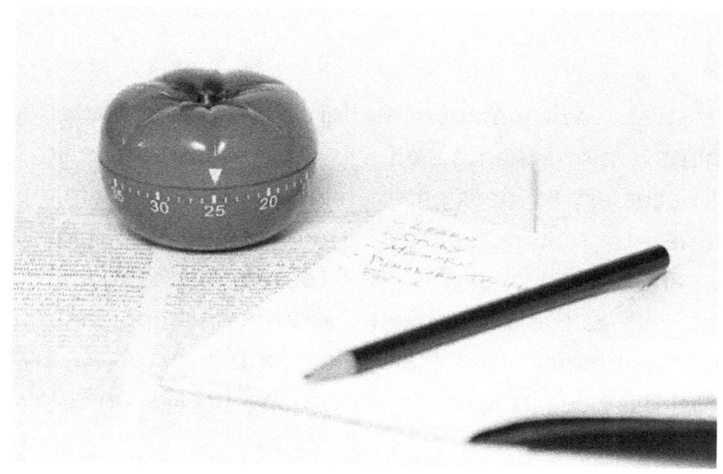

Step 1	📌📋	Pick a Task
Step 2	⏳	Set a 25-Minutes Timer
Step 3	💻✏️	Work On Your Task Until The Time Is Up
Step 4	☕⏱️	Take a 5 Minutes Break
Step 5	🍅	Every 4 Pomodoros, take a longer 15-30 minute break

Thanks to Deborah Kutler "Women With Adhd- A Woman's Journey to Success"

3.2.2: Creating a Vagal-Friendly Workspace

The physical environment of a workspace can significantly influence stress levels. It is helpful to foster a workplace that encourages relaxation and supports vagal health. One must be mindful of ergonomic adjustments to reduce physical strain, the use of plants and natural elements for a calming effect, and the implementation of noise management strategies. Optimizing lighting, temperature, and organization to create a serene and functional work environment is also suggested.

Periodically it would be best to discuss the benefits of occasional changes in the work environment, such as operating in natural light, or varying the location, arrangement of equipment or furniture to refresh the mind and reduce fatigue.

3.2.3: The Role of Social Support at Work

Building a reassuring network within the workplace can be a necessary factor in managing stress. It is important to grow positive relationships with colleagues and create a supportive team environment. Social support at work can lead to a more pleasant work experience, lower stress levels, and consequently more effective vagus nerve function. It is essential to promote effective communication, teamwork and eventual conflict resolution.

There can be no shortage of mentoring programs and peer support, as well as the role of empathy and understanding in building a cohesive work culture.

3.2.4: Balancing Work and Personal Life

It is important to emphasize the importance of establishing clear boundaries between work and home life, especially in the era of remote and hybrid work models.

Also recommended are techniques for disconnecting from work, such as Digital Detox (a period when one decides to unplug from digital devices) and Mindfulness practices.

It is necessary to engage in activities outside of work that nourish the body and soul, such as hobbies, exercise, and quality time with loved ones.

DIGITAL DETOX

Useful tips

Here, then, are some useful tips to start doing digital detox.

- ❖ Reduce smartphone notifications so that only what is really important remains.
- ❖ Limit email synchronization on the smartphone to work hours only.
- ❖ No smartphones at the dinner table and in the bedroom, and if possible, away from the workstation.
- ❖ Set timers and "do not disturb" mode when you decide it is time to stop working and disconnect.
- ❖ Set times to check emails, messages, and to log in first time in the morning and last time in the evening to your various profiles.

Chapter 4: Vagal Health for Parents

4.1: Balancing Parenting with Self-Care

4.1.1: Understanding Parenting Stress and Its Impact on the Vagus Nerve

Parenting, inherently demanding and often relentless, can significantly stress the vagus nerve, which plays a critical role in managing the body's stress response. The unique pressures of parenting—sleepless nights, constant decision-making, and emotional labor—can lead to a persistent activation of the sympathetic nervous system, overwhelming the vagal nerve's capacity to induce calm.

Parental stress specifically affects the vagus nerve, causing symptoms such as increased anxiety, mood fluctuations, digestive problems, and chronic fatigue. It is relevant for parents to recognize these signs as potential indicators of vagal imbalance, emphasizing the interconnection between parental well-being and effective parenting.

4.1.2: Self-Care Strategies for Parents

During parental duties, self-care often takes a back seat, but it is critical to maintain vagal health.

Practical and accessible self-care strategies suitable for time-strapped parents need to be introduced. These are quick and effective techniques such as short mindfulness exercises (Mudra Technique), guided deep breathing sessions (Box Breathing), and simple yoga postures that can be integrated into a busy parenting schedule. These activities are designed to activate the parasympathetic nervous system, thereby improving vagal tone and providing a much-needed respite from the stresses of parenting.

4.1.3: Creating a Self-Care Routine amid Parenting Duties

Making self-care a consistent part of a parent's life requires a roadmap for developing a sustainable daily routine in the chaos of family life.

Time needs to be carved out for personal health, adopting strategies such as waking up a little earlier for a quiet meditation session or joining in a relaxing activity after putting the children to bed.

Let's not forget the value of setting boundaries, such as setting a "me time" during the day, effectively balancing self-care with childcare responsibilities.

4.1.4: The Role of Support Systems

No parent is an island, and a sturdy support system is vital to managing stress and maintaining vaginal health. One must understand the importance of seeking and accepting help from family, friends, and community resources. Sharing responsibilities can significantly relieve parental stress by positively influencing the vagus nerve.

Parents should be encouraged to cultivate a support network, whether through family members or parent groups or professional services, so that they understand the benefits of community connection in enhancing parental well-being and child development.

This holistic approach not only benefits parents but also establishes a more positive and developing environment for their children.

4.2.1: Joint Relaxation and Breathing Exercises

Parent-child bonding can be greatly improved if we engage in activities that also promote vagal health. For example, parents car practice simple but effective relaxation and breathing exercises with their children. These activities not only give a chance to bond and relax together, but also teach children valuable skills for managing their own stress and emotions.

There are exercises suitable for different age groups, such as deep belly breathing, guided visualization (methods to induce relaxation through activation of mental imagination), and gentle stretching. These can be incorporated into daily routines, such as a calming bedtime ritual or a refreshing morning start. By practicing them together, parents and children can simultaneously stimulate the vagus nerves, reducing stress and improving emotional well-being.

Yoga and Mindfulness for Children and Parent

1. ***Yoga's Adaptability for Different Ages and Abilities***:

   - <u>Inclusivity</u>: Yoga is presented as an inclusive activity that can be tailored to various ages, goals, and ability levels. This malleability makes it a practical tool for different settings.

   - <u>Practicality</u>: The ease of practicing yoga with minimal equipment and space requirements is emphasized, making it a practical choice for schools and homes.

2. ***Benefits of Yoga and Mindfulness***:

   - <u>Linked to improved performance</u>: It enhances cognitive functions like focus, concentration, and memory, which are crucial for learning and working.

- <u>Physical Health</u>: Regular yoga practice improves posture, balance, coordination, and body awareness, backing to overall physical fitness.

- <u>Emotional and Social Learning</u>: Yoga fosters an environment of confidence, recreation, and non-competitiveness. It also aids in developing patience, insight, and reduces impulsivity.

3. Implementing Yoga in Educational Settings:

- <u>Creating a Yoga-friendly Environment</u>: Suggestions include designating specific times for yoga, preparing the classroom or home environment, and starting with short sessions to maintain engagement.

- <u>Integration into Daily Routine</u>: The flexibility to incorporate yoga at any time during the school day or home day is highlighted, with an emphasis on aligning yoga practices with the goals of the daily routine.

4. *Yoga Poses Suitable*:

- <u>Simple and Safe Poses</u>: There are lists of easy-to-perform yoga poses that are appropriate, ensuring safety and accessibility.

- <u>Positive Affirmations</u>: Each yoga pose is paired with a positive assertion, like "I am strong" or "I am confident," to help build self-esteem and resilience.

5. *Impact on Social and Emotional Health*:

- <u>Self-Management and Awareness</u>: Yoga and mindfulness practices aid in recognizing and managing their emotions and behaviors. The development of self-regulation and focusing on the present moment is aided by this aspect of yoga.

- <u>Holistic Development</u>: The practices contribute to the holistic development, encompassing physical, emotional, and mental well-being.

Sharing these moments of healthy activity allows parent and child to share a more peaceful and fulfilling life.

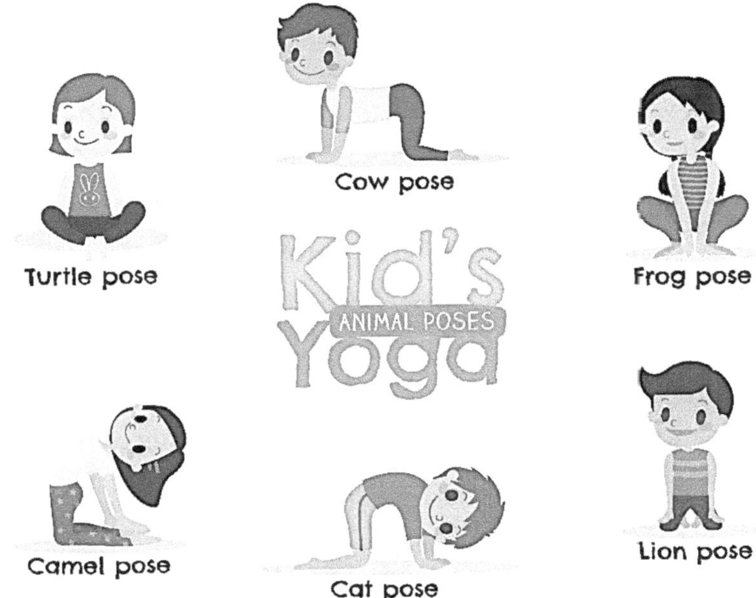

4.2.2: Engaging in Mindful Parent-Child Activities

Mindfulness can be a convincing tool for both parents and children to jointly nurture their vagus nerve.

There are various sporting activities that a family can share and which promote awareness such as "Walking Meditation - Kinhin" and "Nature Walks" in which both the parent and the child can focus on the sensory experiences of the environment; or shared recreational activities like "Mindful Coloring" and "Gardening", where colors, shapes and creativity are the protagonist.

These interests are not only amusing and engaging but also encourage being present "Here & Now", a key aspect of stimulating the vagus nerve. They are practical ideas for embedding mindfulness into everyday parenting tasks, transforming routine interactions into opportunities for enhancing vagal tone.

4.2.3: Nutrition for Vagal Health – A Family Approach

Diet plays an important role in vagus nerve health.

Key factor is a diet rich in anti-inflammatory foods for both parents and children and making nutrition a collaborative and educational family effort. Healthy, family-friendly recipes should be created that are rich in omega-3 fatty acids, probiotics, and any nutrients known to support vagal health.

No less important is to involve children in the cooking process, to make mealtimes a fun and bonding experience and to educate them about the importance of healthy eating.

It would be right for parents to promote healthy eating habits in children to share healthy meals to prevent or reduce vagus nerve inflammation later in life.

4.2.4: The Importance of Play and Laughter

Play and laughter are natural and powerful ways to stimulate the vagus nerve in fact it is relevant to incorporate play and humor into family life. It highlights how involvement in playful activities, from simple games to imaginative play, can be a relieving and joyful experience for both parents and children. Laughter, with its ability to instantly lift the mood and relax the body, is particularly emphasized. There should be no shortage of healthy laughter, funny storytelling, or humorous games in family time. By promoting an atmosphere of joy and play, parents and children can simultaneously improve their vagal health, strengthen their bond, and create lasting, happy memories.

Chapter 5: Diet and the Vagus Nerve

Section 5.1: Foods That Nourish and Heal

A diet rich in specific nutrients can significantly impact the health of the vagus nerve. Below delves into how various foods contribute to the optimal functioning of this crucial nerve. It explains the connection between dietary choices and vagal health, highlighting how certain foods can enhance or hinder the nerve's performance.

5.1.1: Anti-Inflammatory Foods for Vagal Health.

The body's response to inflammation is natural, but when it becomes chronic it can adversely affect various systems, including the vagus nerve, which is critical for managing the body's relaxation response. It is important to incorporate anti-inflammatory foods into one's diet as a strategy to support and improve vagus nerve health.

With several studies, it has been found that there is a direct impact of certain foods that can increase levels of inflammation in the body. The wrong food choice can exacerbate inflammation, leading to decreased vagus nerve function and decreased ability to handle stress and relaxation. Conversely, taking anti-inflammatory foods may help reduce chronic inflammation, potentially improving vagus nerve function.

✓ Omega-3 Fatty Acids: Types and Sources

Special attention is given to omega-3 fatty acids (EPA, DHA and ALA), known for their potent anti-inflammatory properties. Well known are the properties of fatty fish such as salmon, mackerel, and sardines (excellent reserves of EPA and DHA), while flaxseeds, chia seeds, and nuts contain ALA. The benefits of these fatty acids are beneficial to the nervous system, particularly in supporting vagus nerve health.

Note: ***Essential Omega3 Fatty Acid***

EPA: EicosaPentaenoic Acid

DHA: DocosaHexaenoic Acid

ALA: Alpha Linolenic Acid

Nuts and seeds are presented as valuable additions to an anti-inflammatory diet. Almonds, walnuts, flaxseeds, and chia seeds not only provide healthy fats but also contain compounds that help reduce inflammation. In addition, spices like turmeric and ginger are foods from traditional cultures that fight inflammation.

Food Item	Type	Omega-3 Content (per serving)	Notes
Mackerel	Fatty Fish	4,580 mg (3.5 oz)	High in EPA and DHA
Salmon	Fatty Fish	Varies	Popular, widely available
Sardines	Fatty Fish	1,463 mg (1 cup)	Small, oily fish
Herring	Fatty Fish	2,150 mg (3.5 oz)	Often smoked or pickled
Anchovies	Fatty Fish	411 mg (5 anchovies)	Strong flavor
Cod Liver Oil	Fish Oil	2,438 mg (1 tbsp)	High in vitamins D and A
Oysters	Shellfish	329 mg (6 raw oysters)	Rich in zinc and other nutrients
Flaxseeds	Seeds and Nuts	2,350 mg (1 tbsp whole seeds)	Plant-based ALA source
Chia Seeds	Seeds and Nuts	Not specified	High in ALA
Walnuts	Seeds and Nuts	2,570 mg (1 oz)	Good source of ALA

Food Item	Type	Omega-3 Content (per serving)	Notes
Hemp Seeds	Seeds and Nuts	Not specified	Contains ALA
Flaxseed Oil	Plant Oil	High in ALA	Used as an omega-3 supplement
Canola Oil	Plant Oil	Contains omega-3s	Alternative to fish oil
Fortified Foods	Various	Varies	Eggs, dairy, juices
Soybeans	Soy Products	670 mg (1/2 cup dry roasted)	Also high in protein

✓ Antioxidant-Rich Fruits and Vegetables

The discussion then shifts to the function of antioxidants in fighting inflammation. Here the various fruits and vegetables rich in antioxidants and therefore beneficial to vagal health are illustrated. Examples such as berries (blueberries, strawberries, raspberries), green leafy vegetables (spinach, kale) and other vegetables such as broccoli and peppers are included. The importance of consuming a rainbow of fruits and vegetables to maximize the intake of various antioxidants is emphasized.

"Eat the Rainbow & Eat Healthy".

Each color group offers unique health advantages:

1. ***Red Fruits and Vegetables***: Contain lycopene, which aids in stroke prevention, improves heart health, decreases the risk of breast and prostate cancer, and increases brain function. Examples involve tomatoes, beets, cherries, strawberries, red onions, and red peppers.

2. ***Orange and Yellow Fruits and Vegetables***: Rich in carotenoids, these foods reduce heart disease risk, decrease inflammation, boost the immune system, foster healthy skin, and improve vision. Good sources are carrots, winter squash, peaches, yellow peppers, pineapple, bananas, sweet potatoes, mangoes, pumpkins, apricots, and oranges.

3. ***Green Fruits and Vegetables***: Contain isothiocyanates and indoles, which have potential to prevent cancer. They are usually high in potassium, vitamin K, fiber, folic acid, and antioxidants. Examples include spinach, avocados, artichokes, Brussels sprouts, arugula, kiwis, kale, asparagus, fresh green herbs, green tea, and broccoli.

4. ***White and Brown Fruits and Vegetables***: These contain allicin and flavonoids, offering anti-tumor properties, blood pressure reduction and cholesterol, improved bone strength, and decreased risk of stomach cancer. Examples are mushrooms, garlic, cauliflower, onions, and leeks.

5. ***Blue and Purple Fruits and Vegetables***: Packed with antioxidants and anthocyanins, they lower blood pressure, lower the risk of heart disease and stroke, and enhance memory and brain function. Blueberries, blackberries, concord grapes, figs, purple eggplants, cabbage, and plums are good sources.

Rainbow food is not only delicious but also healthful and adds variety to your diet.

5.1.2: Probiotics and Gut Health

✓ Understanding the Gut-Brain Axis and the Vagus Nerve

It's fundamental to remember that there's a complex connection between the gut and brain, known as the gut-brain axis, and the central role of the vagus nerve in this communication system. The gut microbiome – the vast collection of microbes that reside in the intestinal tract – significantly influences both gut health and overall mental well-being. The vagus nerve acts as a two-way communication channel, sending signals from the brain to the gut and vice versa, and this interaction can be influenced by the state of the gut microbiome.

Focusing on probiotics emphasizes their role in maintaining a healthy gut microbiome. Probiotics are valuable bacteria that impact the diversity and balance of gut flora. Important to physical and mental well-being is gut health and, by extension, full vagus nerve function. Keeping a balanced microbiome in check can have a positive impact on vagal tone, leading to improved mood regulation, reduced stress responses, and greater overall mental health.

✓ Sources of Probiotics

Now let's look at a comprehensive overview of natural food sources of probiotics. Included are fermented foods such as Kimchi, Miso, Sauerkraut, Yogurt, Kefir, and kombucha. We note how each of these foods can contribute to gut health and how they are suggested to be incorporated into daily meals.

Probiotics are live microorganisms that, when ingested in appropriate amounts, support health benefits, mostly for the digestive system. The growth of beneficial bacteria is facilitated by the fermentation process, which is why they are commonly found in fermented foods.

Food Item	Description	Key Probiotics	Notes
Yogurt	Fermented milk with live bacteria cultures.	Lactobacillus, Bifidobacterium	Ideal for breakfast, snacks, or smoothies.
Kefir	Drink made from fermented milk, thinner than yogurt.	Yeast and bacteria fusion	
Sauerkraut	Fermented cabbage and vegetables.	Lactobacillus	Choose unpasteurized for live probiotics.

Food Item	Description	Key Probiotics	Notes
Kimchi	Korean dish made from fermented cabbage and vegetables, seasoned with spices.	Lactobacillus	Rich in vitamins and antioxidants.
Miso	Japanese seasoning made by fermenting soybeans with salt and Aspergillus oryzae.		Contributes to healthy gut flora.
Kombucha	Fermented tea drink made by adding bacteria, yeast, and sugar to tea.		Consume in moderation.
Tempeh	Indonesian food made from fermented soybeans.		Firm, protein-rich source of probiotics.
Natto	Japanese food made from fermented soybeans.		High in protein and vitamin K2.

Each of these foods contains different strains and amounts of probiotics, contributing to the diversity of your gut flora. Consuming a variety of these foods can maximize the health benefits for your gut. It's also main to observe that the probiotic content can vary based on factors like the fermentation process and storage conditions.

These foods that are rich in probiotics can be simply added to your diet. For example, you can start your day with Yogurt or kefir, include Sauerkraut or kimchi in your sandwiches or salads, use Miso in soups and dressings, and enjoy kombucha as a refreshing drink.

Having a balanced intestinal microbiome and supporting digestive health are possible through regular consumption of these foods.

The relationship between probiotics, digestion, and the vagus nerve is a fascinating area of study in the field of gut-brain axis research. This relationship highlights the complex dealings between our gut microbiota, digestive health, and nervous system. Here's an in-detailed look at how these elements interact:

Probiotics and Digestion

1. Role of Probiotics in Digestion:

   - The vital role of maintaining gut health is played by probiotics, the beneficial bacteria found in fermented foodstuffs and supplements.

   - They aid in decomposing food, absorbing nutrients, and can help balance the gut microbiota, which is vital for efficient digestion.

   - By enhancing the gut flora, probiotics contribute to a more robust intestinal lining, reducing the likelihood of harmful bacteria and toxins passing into the bloodstream (a phenomenon known as "leaky gut").

2. Alleviating Digestive Issues:

   - Regular intake of probiotics has been linked to alleviation of common gastrointestinal problems like bloating, gas, and irregular bowel movements.

   - They help in the management of illnesses like Irritable Bowel Syndrome (IBS), Inflammatory Bowel Disease (IBD), and diarrhea, particularly antibiotic-associated diarrhea.

Impact on the Vagus Nerve

1. Vagus Nerve Overview:

   - The vagus nerve is a fundamental branch of the parasympathetic nervous system and acts a vital role in regulating the digestive system.

- It controls mechanisms like the release of digestive enzymes, gut motility, and the secretion of certain hormones related to digestion and appetite.

2. Probiotics and Vagal Stimulation:

- Improved digestion facilitated by a healthy gut microbiome can positively influence the vagus nerve's function.

- Probiotics can indirectly stimulate the vagus nerve by enhancing gut health. A well-functioning digestive system sends positive signals to the brain via the vagus nerve, promoting a state of homeostasis and well-being.

- Some studies recommend that certain probiotic strains can directly impact the vagus nerve. For instance, Lactobacillus strains have been shown to have a direct effect on the vagus nerve, influencing mood and anxiety levels, which are often regulated through the gut-brain axis.

3. Feedback Loop:

- There's a feedback loop between the gut and the brain, through the vagus nerve. A healthy gut can lead to more effective vagal signaling, which in turn can further enhance digestive processes and overall gut health.

- This relationship is bidirectional. Just as a healthy gut can positively influence the vagus nerve, stress, or anxiety, which affect the nervous system, can also impact gut health, demonstrating the interconnectedness of these systems.

The correlation between probiotics, digestion, and the vagus nerve is proof of the complexity of the human body and the interconnectedness of our systems.

✓ Integrating Probiotic Foods into a Healthy Diet

Integrating probiotic-rich foods into your daily diet is a key strategy for maintaining gut health, which can have a profound impact on overall well-being, including optimal vagal function. Here are practical tips and ideas for adding these foods into meals and snacks, catering to diverse tastes and dietary preferences:

Breakfast Ideas

1. Yogurt Parfaits: Layer Greek yogurt with fruits, nuts, and a touch of honey. Yogurt is a versatile probiotic food that can be enjoyed in many ways.

2. Kefir Smoothies: Blend kefir with your choice of fruits, greens, and seeds for a nutritious start to your day.

3. Probiotic Oats: Stir in a spoonful of natural yogurt into your oatmeal and top with fresh berries.

Lunch Ideas

1. Sauerkraut or Kimchi as a Side: Add these fermented vegetables to your sandwiches, wraps, or salads. They add a tangy flavor and are rich in probiotics.

2. Miso Soup: A light and healthy starter, it can be an excellent extra to your lunch.

Dinner Ideas

1. Tempeh or Natto Dishes: Use these fermented soy products as the main protein in your meals. They can be grilled, sautéed, or inserted to stir-fries.

2. Kombucha Marinades: Use kombucha as a base for marinades to add a unique flavor to your meats or vegetables.

Snack Ideas

1. Cheese and Crackers: Certain cheeses like Gouda, Cheddar, and Swiss contain probiotics. Combine with wholegrain crackers to create an enjoyable snack.

2. Pickled Vegetables: Snack on pickled cucumbers, carrots, or other vegetables for a probiotic boost.

Dessert Ideas

1. Frozen Yogurt: Opt for natural, unsweetened frozen yogurt topped with fruits.

2. Probiotic Fruit Popsicles: Blend kefir with fruits and freeze them in popsicle molds.

Tips for Consistency and Variety

1. Daily Probiotic Intake: Aim to include at least one probiotic-rich food in your diet every day.

2. Diverse Sources: Rotate different probiotic foods to benefit from various strains of beneficial bacteria.

3. Pair with Prebiotics: Combine probiotic foods with prebiotic-rich foods like garlic, onions, bananas, or oats to enhance their benefits.

4. Homemade Ferments: Consider making your own yogurt, kefir, or fermented vegetables to ensure quality and potency of probiotics.

5. Mindful of Pasteurization: Remember that pasteurization can kill beneficial bacteria, so opt for unpasteurized versions when safe and possible.

Importance of Consistency

- Regular consumption of probiotic foods contributes to a balanced gut microbiome.
- A healthy gut microbiome supports efficient digestion, immune function, and can positively influence vagal nerve activity.
- To reduce the risk of inflammation and other intestinal problems, it's best to consume probiotics regularly to maintain the integrity of the intestinal lining.

Incorporating probiotic foods into your diet isn't just about adding new ingredients; it's about creating a balanced and sustainable eating habit that supports your gut health. By regularly consuming a variety of probiotic-rich foods, you can ensure a healthy gut microbiome, which is crucial for overall health, including optimal function of the vagus nerve. Remember, the key is consistency and variety to reap the full benefits of probiotics.

✓ Supplementing with Probiotics

For those who are unable to obtain sufficient probiotics from their diet, it is recommended that they consult their physician who will arrange for possible prescription of effective probiotic supplements.

5.1.3: Hydration and the Vagus Nerve

✓ Water's Role in Vagal Health

Adequate hydration of the body, and in particular of the vagus nerve, is of paramount importance in order to regulate many bodily processes.

"Water's Role in Vagal Health" is a topic that delves into the critical importance of hydration for the optimal functioning of the vagus nerve, a key part of the parasympathetic nervous system. The vagus nerve has a significant role in controlling different bodily functions, such as heart rate, digestion, and immune response. Here's an in-depth look at how right hydration supports vagal health:

Hydration and Electrolyte Balance

1. Electrolytes and Nerve Function:

   - Electrolytes such as calcium, potassium, sodium, and magnesium are crucial for nerve signal transmission.

   - The vagus nerve, like other nerves, relies on these electrolytes to carry electrical signals throughout the body.

- Proper hydration ensures that these electrolytes are maintained at optimal levels, facilitating efficient nerve function.

2. Impact of Dehydration:

   - Dehydration can lead to an imbalance in electrolytes, disrupting the normal function of nerves, including the vagus nerve.

   - This imbalance can impair the vagus nerve's ability to effectively transmit signals, potentially leading to reduced function in the systems it regulates.

Water Intake, Blood Pressure, and Heart Rate

1. Regulation of Blood Pressure:

   - Sufficient hydration helps preserve blood volume, which is crucial for stable blood pressure.

   - Dehydration can lead to low blood volume (hypovolemia), causing blood pressure to drop, which may trigger compensatory mechanisms that the vagus nerve helps to regulate.

2. Influence on Heart Rate:

   - The vagus nerve is instrumental in controlling heart rate. Hydration status can influence heart rate and its variability.

   - Proper hydration supports the vagus nerve in maintaining a normal heart rate, while dehydration can lead to increased heart rate and reduced vagal tone.

Hydration and Digestive Health

1. Vagal Stimulation in Digestion:

   - The vagus nerve is involved in initiating digestive processes. Adequate hydration aids in digestion, indirectly supporting the vagal activity.

   - Water is essential for the proper function of the gastrointestinal tract, facilitating the movement of food and absorption of nutrients.

Practical Tips for Adequate Hydration

1. Regular Water Intake:

   - Aim for regular, consistent water intake throughout the day. Although the typical guideline is 8-10 glasses of water per day, individual needs may differ.

   - Include foods with elevated water content, like fruits and vegetables, in your nutritional regime.

2. Monitoring Hydration Levels:

   - Pay attention to symptoms of dehydration, like dry mouth, fatigue, and dark urine.

   - Use thirst as a guide, but don't wait for it to drink water, as thirst can be a late sign of dehydration.

3. Balanced Electrolyte Intake:

   - Along with water, ensure a balanced intake of electrolytes, especially if you are engaged in activities that cause significant sweating.

   ✓ Signs of Dehydration and Its Impact on the Vagus Nerve.

To maintain vagal health, it is essential to recognize signs of dehydration.

Symptoms of Dehydration	Impact on Vagus Nerve	Proactive Steps for Prevention
Fatigue and Weakness	Heightened stress response, reducing vagal tone	Regular fluid intake, monitor physical changes
Dizziness and Lightheadedness	Cardiovascular strain due to lower blood pressure	Adequate water consumption, mindful activity planning
Dry Mouth and Thirst	Impaired digestive functions, reduced saliva production	Consistent water consumption, include high water content foods
Decreased Urine Output	Potential digestive discomfort and constipation	Monitor urine color and frequency, ensure electrolyte balance
Headaches	Increased stress levels, anxiety	Regular hydration, monitor for early signs of dehydration
Cognitive Impairment	Reduced nutrient absorption, digestive issues	Adequate hydration, dietary considerations for water-rich foods

✓ Hydrating Beverages for Vagal Health

Although water is the primary source of hydration, other beverages can also aid in hydrating the body and supporting the vagus nerve. Herbal teas are appreciated for their calming properties and can indirectly promote vagal function by inducing relaxation. However, it is important to limit the consumption of beverages that can lead to dehydration or increased stress response, such as those high in caffeine or alcohol.

✓ Practical Tips for Maintaining Optimal Hydration

Proper hydration is essential for various bodily functions, including preserving the balance of bodily fluids, facilitating digestion, and regulating body temperature. Here are some in-depth practical tips and strategies to help integrate optimal hydration into your daily routine:

Increasing Water Intake

1. <u>Begin your day with water</u>: start with a glass of water every morning, after a night of fasting.

2. <u>Carry a Reusable Water Bottle</u>: Having water in hand always makes it easier to drink regularly throughout the day.

3. <u>Set Regular Reminders</u>: Make sure to drink water at regular intervals by using phone alarms or apps.

4. <u>Hydrate Before, During, and After Exercise</u>: Restore the fluids that have been lost due to sweat during physical activity.

5. <u>Drink Water with Every Meal</u>: Establish a routine of drinking water before, during, and after meals.

Incorporating Hydrating Foods

1. <u>Eat Water-Rich Fruits and Vegetables</u>: Foods like cucumbers, tomatoes, oranges, watermelon, and berries are high in water content.

2. <u>Include Soups and Broths in Your Diet</u>: These can be hydrating and also a good source of nutrients.

3. <u>Opt for Smoothies</u>: Blend fruits and vegetables with water or coconut water for a hydrating snack.

Creating Hydration Habits

1. _Establish a Routine_: Link drinking water with daily activities like after waking up, before meals, and before bedtime.

2. _Track Your Intake_: Use a journal or an app to keep track of how much water you drink each day.

3. _Understand Your Individual Needs_: Factors like body weight, climate, activity level, and health conditions affect hydration needs.

Making Water Intake Appealing

1. _Infuse Water with Fruits or Herbs_: Add slices of lemon, lime, cucumber, or mint to enhance the flavor of water.

2. _Try Sparkling Water_: If you prefer a fizzy drink, sparkling water can be a good alternative to soda.

3. _Experiment with Herbal Teas_: Unsweetened herbal teas can be a hydrating, caffeine-free option.

Recognizing Personal Hydration Cues

1. _Listen to Your Body_: Thirst is an obvious sign of dehydration, but it is not wise to wait until you are thirsty to drink.

2. _Monitor Urine Color_: Light, pale-yellow urine typically indicates proper hydration, while dark urine suggests a need for more fluids.

3. _Be Aware of Other Dehydration Signs_: Dry skin, fatigue, and headaches can also suggest that you need to drink more water.

✓ Impact of Certain Foods on the Vagus Nerve

After highlighting how hydration is a key part of the nervous system, we now go on to understand how certain foods can have a negative impact on the vagus nerve and overall health. Although the focus is on what should be included in a diet for vagal health, it is equally important to understand what to avoid. In an uncontrolled diet there are certain foods that can exacerbate inflammation, disrupt gut health, and impair vagus nerve function, causing a range of problems, from increased stress response to digestive problems.

✓ Pro-Inflammatory Foods

Chronic inflammation is linked to various health issues, including impaired vagal health, and can be influenced significantly by what we eat. Here's an in-depth look at foods with pro-inflammatory properties:

Types of Pro-Inflammatory Foods

> Processed Meats: Sausages, bacon, and deli meats are elevated in saturated fats and additives that can trigger inflammation.
> Fried Foods: Foods that are deep-fried, like French-fries and fried chicken, frequently have trans fats, which are known to promote inflammation.
> Refined Carbohydrates: Products with refined flour (White bread, pastries, etc.) can strengthen inflammation.
> Sugary Beverages: Soft drinks and other sweetened drinks are high in added sugars, contributing to systemic inflammation.
> Excessive Alcohol: High consumption of alcohol can lead to inflammation and damage to body tissues.

Impact on Systemic Inflammation

- ➢ <u>Saturated and Trans Fats</u>: These fats can activate inflammatory pathways and increase the production of pro-inflammatory cytokines.
- ➢ <u>High Glycemic Index Foods</u>: Foods that rapidly increase blood sugar levels can spur inflammation by causing an overproduction of insulin.
- ➢ <u>Imbalance of Omega-6 to Omega-3 Fatty Acids</u>: A diet high in omega-6 fatty acids (found in many processed foods) and low in omega-3s can contribute to inflammation.

Advanced Glycation End Products (AGEs)

- ➢ <u>Formation of AGEs</u>: AGEs are formed when protein or fat combine with sugar in the bloodstream, a process accelerated during high-temperature cooking (like grilling, frying, or roasting).
- ➢ <u>Role in Inflammation</u>: AGEs can promote oxidative stress and inflammation by damaging cells and tissues in the body.
- ➢ <u>Dietary Sources of AGEs</u>: Foods high in protein and fat are more likely to form AGEs when cooked at high temperatures.

Impact on Vagal Health

- ➢ <u>Systemic Inflammation and the Vagus Nerve</u>: Chronic inflammation can negatively impact the vagus nerve, which plays a key role in regulating inflammation and maintaining homeostasis in the body.
- ➢ <u>Impaired Gut Health</u>: Pro-inflammatory foods can disrupt the gut microbiome, indirectly affecting vagal tone due to the gut-brain axis connection.

Foods high in sugar can cause rapid spikes in blood sugar levels. These spikes are not just a concern for blood sugar management but also for overall inflammation in the body. When blood sugar levels rise sharply, the body responds by releasing insulin in large amounts, a process that, over time, can develop insulin resistance, a key cause in type 2 diabetes and obesity. This state of elevated blood sugar and insulin resistance is closely linked to increased inflammation, which can put a strain on various bodily systems, including the vagus nerve.

Refined carbohydrates, found in foods like white bread, pastries, and many processed snacks, contribute to these issues in a similar way. A rapid increase in blood sugar levels occurs due to the high glycemic index of these foods. Unlike whole grains, refined carbs lack fiber, which is essential for gut health. Fiber plays a fundamental role in maintaining a healthy gut microbiome and promoting regular bowel movements, both of which are important for optimal vagal function. A diet deficient in fiber can lead to an imbalance in gut bacteria and, consequently, gut inflammation. This disruption in gut health can negatively impact the vagus nerve, as there is a strong connection between the gut and the brain, often described as the gut-brain axis.

✓ Artificial Additives and Preservatives

In today's food industry, artificial additives and preservatives are widely used to enhance flavor, appearance, and shelf life of food products. However, their impact on health, particularly on the gut microbiome and the vagus nerve, is a growing concern.

Artificial additives, which include colorants, flavor enhancers, and artificial sweeteners, along with preservatives like sodium benzoate and sulfites, can disrupt the delicate balance of the gut microbiome. A complex ecosystem of bacteria and other microorganisms known as the gut microbiome plays a vital role in digestion, immune function, and mental health. When this balance is disturbed, it can lead to a series of issues, including inflammation, digestive problems, and a weakened immune response. This disruption is particularly concerning because of the gut-brain axis, a communication network that links the gut and the brain, of which the vagus nerve is a key component.

The vagus nerve, responsible for regulating many automatic functions in the body, can be affected by changes in the gut microbiome. An imbalance in gut bacteria, potentially caused by artificial additives and preservatives, can lead to decreased vagal tone, meaning the nerve becomes less efficient at sending and receiving signals. This can manifest in various symptoms, such as poor digestion, irregular heart rate, and an impaired ability to manage stress.

Given these potential impacts, it is advisable for people:

- To be aware of their consumption of foods containing artificial additives and preservatives.
- Reading food labels carefully is a good practice to identify and limit the consumption of these chemicals.
- Choosing for whole, unprocessed foods as much as possible is another effective strategy. Whole foods, such as fruits, vegetables, whole grains, and lean proteins, are free from artificial additives and preservatives and offer a range of nutrients that support gut health and overall well-being.
- By making educated decisions about the foods we consume, we can help maintain the health of our gut microbiome and ensure the optimal functioning of the vagus nerve, contributing to better health overall.

✓ Caffeine and Alcohol

The consequences of caffeine and alcohol on the vagus nerve are often discussed. Moderate caffeine consumption can be beneficial for a healthy diet, but excessive consumption can over-stimulate the nervous system, including the vagus nerve, leading to heightened stress responses. Similarly, the section outlines how excessive alcohol consumption can negatively impact the gut-brain axis, interfere with sleep patterns, and ultimately impair vagal function.

P.s.: We recommend Olivia Jane Fisher's Book

The Anti-Inflammatory Diet Cookbook for Beginners

5.2: Creating a Vagus-Healthy Meal Plan

Section 5.2.1: Meal Planning for Vagal Health

1) Introduction to Meal Planning for Vagal Health

A diet that supports vagal health is one that minimizes inflammation, balances the gut microbiome, and ensures adequate hydration.

A well-structured meal plan is more than just a tool for healthy eating; it's a strategic approach to consistently incorporate specific types of foods that benefit the vagus nerve. By planning meals in advance, individuals can ensure they are regularly consuming anti-inflammatory foods, probiotics, and maintaining proper hydration, all of which are crucial for optimal vagal function.

Anti-inflammatory foods, corresponding leafy greens, berries, nuts, and fatty fish like salmon, contain nutrients that help reduce systemic inflammation, a condition that can adversely affect the vagus nerve. Including these foods in a meal plan can help mitigate inflammation and support the overall health of the nervous system.

As previously stated, probiotics, which are present in fermented foods such as yogurt, kefir, sauerkraut, and kimchi, are vital for preserving a healthy intestinal microbiome. The gut-brain axis, which involves direct and indirect pathways between the gut and the brain, highlights the importance of gut health in regulating the function of the vagus nerve. A meal plan that includes a variety of probiotic-rich foods can help ensure a balanced gut microbiome, which in turn supports the health of the vagus nerve.

In summary, meal planning for vagal health involves a conscious effort to include foods and beverages that support the functioning of the vagus nerve. This approach not only simplifies the process of eating healthily but also ensures a consistent intake of key nutrients and probiotics, along with adequate hydration. Such a plan can be instrumental in systematically enhancing vagal health, contributing to improved overall well-being.

1.a. Fundamentals of a Vagus-Healthy Diet

A diet that supports the health of this nerve is multifaceted, focusing on anti-inflammatory foods, probiotics, adequate hydration, and a balanced intake of macronutrients. We recall below the basic concepts.

At the core of a vagus-healthy diet is the emphasis on anti-inflammatory foods. Chronic inflammation can impair the role of the vagus nerve. Incorporating a variety of foods rich in antioxidants and anti-inflammatory compounds is crucial. These include leafy greens, berries, nuts, seeds, and fatty fish like salmon. These foods provide essential nutrients that help mitigate inflammation throughout the body, thereby supporting the health of the vagus nerve.

Probiotics are another cornerstone of this diet. Found in fermented foods, probiotics help keep a healthy gut microbiome. The gut-brain axis is significantly influenced by the state of the gut flora. A balanced microbiome aids in efficient digestion, nutrient absorption, and immune function, all of which are regulated by the vagus nerve.

Adequate water intake ensures the maintenance of electrolyte balance, crucial for nerve signal transmission. This balance is vital for the correct functioning of the vagus nerve, which in turn regulates many bodily processes. Including hydrating foods in the diet, along with regular water consumption, is essential for maintaining this balance.

The balance of macronutrients - carbohydrates, proteins, and fats - is also key in a vagus-healthy diet. Carbohydrates should primarily come from high-fiber, whole-food sources such as whole grains, fruits, and vegetables. These foods provide the necessary fiber for gut health, which is closely linked to the function of the vagus nerve. Healthy fats, particularly omega-3 fatty acids found in fish, flaxseeds, and walnuts, are important for reducing inflammation and supporting brain health, which is interconnected with the function of the vagus nerve. Lean proteins, from sources like poultry, fish, legumes, and tofu, provide the essential building blocks for the body's tissues and enzymes, aiding in the overall support of bodily functions controlled by the vagus nerve.

1.b. Creating a Balanced Meal Plan

Creating a balanced meal plan for those with vagus nerve inflammation involves incorporating foods that support vagal health. This plan will focus on anti-inflammatory foods, probiotics, hydration, and a balance of macronutrients. Here's a sample meal plan:

Breakfast

- **Option 1**: Oatmeal made with almond milk, topped with fresh berries (rich in antioxidants), chia seeds (high in omega-3), and a dollop of Greek yogurt (probiotic).

- **Option 2**: Smoothie with spinach, banana, flaxseed oil (omega-3 source), kefir (probiotic), and a scoop of protein powder.

Mid-Morning Snack

- **Option 1**: A small bowl of mixed nuts and seeds.

- **Option 2**: Sliced apple with almond butter.

Lunch

- ***Option 1***: Grilled salmon salad with mixed greens, avocado (healthy fats), cherry tomatoes, and a vinaigrette dressing.

- ***Option 2***: Whole-grain wrap filled with turkey breast, mixed salad leaves, cucumber, and hummus.

Afternoon Snack

- ***Option 1***: Carrot and cucumber sticks with a yogurt-based dip.

- ***Option 2***: A piece of fruit (like an orange or pear) and a handful of berries.

Dinner

- ***Option 1***: Stir-fried chicken with broccoli, bell peppers, and brown rice. Use ginger and garlic for flavor (anti-inflammatory).

- ***Option 2***: Baked cod with a side of quinoa and steamed asparagus. Drizzle with olive oil (healthy fat) and lemon.

Evening Snack

- ***Option 1***: A small bowl of mixed berries with a sprinkle of ground flaxseed.

- ***Option 2***: A cup of herbal tea (like chamomile) and a few squares of dark chocolate (at least 70% cocoa).

Hydration

- Ensure regular water intake throughout the day. Aim for at least 8 glasses of water.

- Herbal teas and infused water (for example with cucumber, lemon, or mint) are good options.

Personalization Tips

- *Vegetarian/Vegan*: Replace animal proteins with plant-based alternatives (tofu, tempeh, and legumes).

- *Gluten-Free*: Opt for gluten-free grains such as quinoa, gluten-free oats and buckwheat.

- *Dairy-Free*: Use plant-based yogurt and milk alternatives, and dairy-free probiotic supplements if needed.

This meal plan is designed to provide a balanced intake of nutrients that support vagal health, with a focus on anti-inflammatory foods, probiotics, and hydration. It's important to adjust the plan according to individual dietary needs and preferences. Regular consultation with a healthcare provider or a dietitian is recommended to ensure the meal plan meets all nutritional requirements and supports overall health, especially for those with specific health conditions like vagus nerve inflammation.

1.c. Strategies for Effective Meal Planning

Effective meal planning is not just about choosing the right foods; it's also about creating a system that fits seamlessly into one's lifestyle, ensuring consistency and ease.

One key strategy is <u>Batch cooking.</u> This involves preparing large quantities of certain staples or entire meals at the beginning of the week or on a designated cooking day. Saving time and reducing stress of daily meal preparation can be achieved by batch cooking. For example, cooking a large batch of brown rice, grilling several chicken breasts, or roasting a variety of vegetables can provide the base for multiple meals throughout the week. These can be quickly assembled into different combinations, ensuring variety while maintaining a focus on vagal-healthy foods.

Using a shopping list is another crucial strategy. A well-thought-out shopping list, based on the meal plan for the week, ensures that all necessary ingredients are purchased in one go, reducing the frequency of shopping trips and the temptation to buy unhealthy, impulsive choices. This list should focus on health-promoting ingredients that support the vagus nerve, such as leafy greens, fruits rich in antioxidants, sources of healthy fats like avocados and nuts, lean proteins, and fermented foods rich in probiotics.

Planning for snacks is equally important. Snacks are often where impulsive and unhealthy eating habits can creep in. By planning healthy snacks, such as cut vegetables with hummus, Greek yogurt with fruit, or a handful of nuts, one can avoid reaching for processed or high-sugar options. Having these healthier alternatives readily available can greatly aid in sticking to a vagus-healthy diet.

Adapting meal plans for busy schedules is crucial. Not everyone has the time for extensive meal preparation. For those with hectic lifestyles, the focus should be on quick and healthy meals. This can include simple stir-fries that combine a protein source with an array of vegetables, quick salads with canned beans or fish, or smoothies that can be prepared in minutes. The use of healthy pre-prepared or frozen ingredients can also be a time-saving strategy.

1.d. Incorporating Flexibility and Variety

Flexibility in meal planning is crucial. It's important to recognize that life is unpredictable and that strict adherence to a meal plan may not always be feasible. Allowing room for adjustments based on time constraints, availability of ingredients, or simply one's mood, can make the process more sustainable in the long run. For instance, if a planned ingredient is not available, knowing how to substitute it with something similar can keep the meal both nutritious and interesting.

Variety is another key aspect. Eating the same foods repeatedly can become tedious and may lead to a lack of essential nutrients. Experimenting with new recipes and ingredients not only broadens the nutritional profile of the diet but also keeps the excitement alive in cooking and eating. Trying out different cuisines, cooking methods, and flavor combinations can transform meal preparation into a creative and enjoyable activity.

Seasonal produce plays a significant role in adding variety to meals. Each season offers a unique array of fruits and vegetables. Incorporating these seasonal items into the diet ensures that meals are fresh, nutrient-dense, and aligned with the body's seasonal needs. It also supports local farming and is environmentally sustainable.

Making meal planning for vagal health enjoyable is essential. It shouldn't feel like a strict regimen but rather a flexible and enjoyable part of one's lifestyle. This approach can include themed meal nights, like "Taco Tuesday" or "Stir-Fry Saturday," to add an element of fun and anticipation. It can also involve family or friends in the meal planning and preparation process, making it a shared and social activity.

1.e Meal Preparation Techniques and Vagal Health

The importance of cooking techniques lies in determining the retention of nutrients in food. Methods like steaming or grilling are often recommended for preserving the integrity of vitamins and minerals in vegetables and proteins. Steaming is particularly effective for vegetables, as it minimizes nutrient loss, which can be more pronounced in methods that involve water, such as boiling. Grilling, on the other hand, can be a healthy way to prepare proteins like fish or chicken, as it requires minimal oil and can enhance flavor without significantly reducing nutrient content.

Conversely, high-heat methods like deep-frying are generally advised to be minimized. While these methods can add appealing flavors and textures, they can also lead to the loss of beneficial nutrients and the formation of harmful compounds, including tranny fats and Advanced Glycation end Products (AGEs). Inflammation and oxidative stress may be exacerbated by these compounds, potentially impacting the vagus nerve's function.

The role of mindful eating practices is another crucial aspect of this topic.

Eating consciously means paying full attention to the eating experience and enjoying each bite. It encourages a more contemplative and slow approach to eating meals, which can have several benefits for digestion and vagal health. By eating mindfully, individuals can better tune into their body's hunger and fullness cues, helping in controlling portions and decrease the risk of overeating. This practice can also enhance digestion, as it promotes thorough chewing and allows more time for the digestive process to begin in the mouth.

Moreover, mindful eating can positively influence the vagus nerve. The act of eating slowly and attentively can stimulate the vagus nerve, enhancing its role in regulating digestion and promoting a state of calm. This can be especially useful for people with digestive problems, as a well-functioning vagus nerve is essential for efficient digestive processes.

5.2.2: Mindful Eating Practices

1. Introduction to Mindful Eating

Conscious eating is a method that requires complete focus on the sensations of eating and drinking, both internal and external to the body. It encourages individuals to savor each bite, to be fully engaged with the act of eating, without distraction or haste.

Observing the colors, smells, textures, flavors, temperatures, and even sounds of our meals is what this practice involves. Acknowledging the signs of hunger and satiety in the body is also important, understanding when to start and stop eating based on these signals.

By eating slowly and chewing thoroughly, individuals can aid the mechanical breakdown of food and the absorption of nutrients, facilitating smoother digestion. This slower, more deliberate process of eating can lead to better digestion and nutrient absorption, and by extension, support the health of the vagus nerve.

Furthermore, mindful eating is presented as a method to reduce stress. In today's fast-paced world, meals are frequently eaten quickly or in a distracted state. This practice of eating mindfully helps to create a moment of calm in the day, allowing the body to focus on the task of eating and digesting. By reducing stress and promoting a state of relaxation while eating, mindful eating can positively influence the vagus nerve, known for its role in the parasympathetic nervous system, often referred to as the "rest and digest" system.

2. The Connection Between Mindful Eating and Vagal Health

Mindful eating, characterized by eating in a calm and attentive state, is shown to actively engage the parasympathetic nervous system, often referred to as the "rest and digest" system.

When eating mindfully, Individuals are more likely to take their time while eating and chew their food thoroughly, which facilitates the mechanical breakdown of food and eases the digestive process. This slower, more deliberate approach to eating allows the vagus nerve to efficiently regulate the digestive tract's activities, enhancing the absorption of nutrients and reducing the likelihood of common gastrointestinal issues such as bloating, indigestion, and discomfort.

Likewise, the practice of mindful eating is closely linked to the prevention of overeating. Being very careful about the body's hunger and fullness cues, people who eat mindfully are better capable of controlling their food intake. So, not only does this only promote weight management, but also avoids straining of the digestive system, as often happens when overeating.

Excessive consumption of food can lead to a host of digestive problems, which can in turn impact the vagus nerve's ability to function optimally. By promoting a more balanced approach to eating, mindful eating supports the health of the vagus nerve.

3. *Principles of Mindful Eating*

Principle	Description
Eating Slowly	Take time with each bite, chew thoroughly, and do not rush the meal.
Savoring Each Bite	Focus on the sensory experience of eating, embracing the taste, texture, and aroma of the food.
Paying Attention	Make meals a time to be fully present and avoid distractions like TV or smartphones.
Listening to Hunger Cues	Eat when you feel physiological hunger, rather than due to external cues or emotional reasons.
Recognizing Fullness	Stop eating when you are satisfied, not when your plate is empty.
Responding to Body's Needs	Choose foods that nourish and satisfy your body, take note of the sensations of various foods.
Mindful Selection of Food	Choose foods that are both liking to you and beneficial to your body.
Appreciating Your Food	Take a moment to convey gratitude for your meal and consider its origins and preparation.

6.1: Types of Exercises Beneficial for the Vagus Nerve

The connection between exercise and vagal tone is a fascinating and crucial aspect of understanding how physical activity influences overall health, particularly the function of the vagus nerve and the parasympathetic nervous system.

6.1.a Overview of the Vagus Nerve and Parasympathetic System.

- *Vagus Nerve Function*: The vagus nerve is a key element of the parasympathetic nervous system, which is often referred to as the "rest and digest" system. It helps to slow down the heart rate, regulate digestion, and promote a state of calm and relaxation in the body.
- *Vagal Tone*: It indicates the activity level of the vagus nerve. Higher vagal tone is associated with a better ability to relax after stress and is often linked to a healthier cardiovascular state, better glucose regulation, and reduced risk of inflammation-related diseases.

6.1.b Influence of Different Types of Exercise on the Vagus Nerve.

<u>Cardiovascular Exercise</u>

- *Effect on Heart Rate Variability (HRV)*: Cardiovascular exercises like running, cycling, and swimming increase heart rate and respiratory rate initially but can lead to an increase in heart rate variability (HRV) over time. Higher HRV is a marker of good vagal tone.
- *Long-term Benefits*: Regular aerobic exercise can enhance the body's ability to manage stress, partly due to the improved efficiency and resilience of the cardiovascular system supported by a well-functioning vagus nerve.

Strength Training

- ◆ *Muscle Activation and Relaxation*: Strength training exercises require controlled muscle contraction and relaxation, which can positively affect the nervous system. The focus and discipline involved in strength training can also induce a state of mindful presence, reducing stress and stimulating the parasympathetic response.
- ◆ *Hormonal Response*: Strength training regulates stress hormones like cortisol, which, when elevated, can negatively affect the vagus nerve. By managing these hormonal levels, strength training supports parasympathetic activity.

Flexibility and Mobility Exercises

- ◆ Impact on Stress and Tension: Flexibility exercises, such as stretching and mobility routines, can help relieve physical tension, a common physical manifestation of stress. Reduced muscle tension can signal the brain to promote a parasympathetic response.
- ◆ Yoga and Pilates: Practices like yoga and Pilates combine flexibility with deep breathing and mindful movement, directly stimulating the vagus nerve and enhancing its tone.

Relaxation and Mind-Body Exercises

- ◆ Direct Stimulation of the Vagus Nerve: Exercises like yoga, tai chi, and qigong, which emphasize relaxation and breath control, directly stimulate the vagus nerve. These practices often involve diaphragmatic breathing, which activates the parasympathetic response.
- ◆ Reducing Mental Stress: Relaxation exercises help in reducing mental stress and anxiety, which in turn prevents the overstimulation of the sympathetic nervous system, allowing the

parasympathetic system, including the vagus nerve, to operate more effectively.

Conclusion: Exercise influences vagal tone by enhancing the body's ability to shift between the sympathetic and parasympathetic states efficiently, a critical aspect of maintaining health and resilience. Different types of exercise contribute in varied ways to this balance, underscoring the importance of a diverse and balanced exercise regimen for optimal vagal health.

6.2 Specific Exercises for Enhancing Vagal Tone

Specific exercises designed to enhance vagal tone focus on stimulating the parasympathetic nervous system, thereby improving the function of the vagus nerve. These exercises generally encourage relaxation, stress reduction, and a balanced autonomic nervous system. Here are some key examples:

1. **Deep Breathing Exercises**

- *Diaphragmatic Breathing (Belly Breathing)*: Involves deep, slow breathing that engages the diaphragm, encouraging full oxygen exchange, promoting relaxation and stimulating the vagus nerve.

- *4-7-8 Breathing*: It is a simple yet powerful breathing technique that helps calm the nervous system, reduce stress and improve sleep. How to do it: Breathe in for 4 seconds, hold for 7 seconds, and exhale for 8 seconds.

- *Lion's Breath* is a yogic breathing technique that involves forceful exhalation with a wide-open mouth, extended tongue, and a roaring sound. It is used to relieve tension, stimulate and clear the throat chakra, and enhance energy flow.

- *"Breath of Fire" - Kapalabhati Pranayama*: It is a yogic breathing technique that combines rapid, forceful exhalations with passive inhalations. A typical session might include one to three rounds, each lasting about 20 to 30 breaths, with a short pause in between.

Let's learn more about the Breath of Fire.

Derived from Sanskrit, *kapala* means "skull," and *bhati* means "light" or "shining." This pranayama technique is thought to cleanse the respiratory system and energize the mind, often described as bringing "clarity to the skull."

In practice, Kapalabhati begins with a deep inhale followed by a series of short, quick exhales through the nose, driven by forceful contractions of the abdominal muscles. These active exhalations are often compared to a bellows effect, with the passive inhale following naturally between each exhale.

Physically, Kapalabhati helps cleanse the respiratory system by expelling stale air, allowing fresh oxygen to fill the lungs. The technique strengthens the diaphragm and abdominal muscles, improves digestion, and enhances lung capacity. Mentally, it is known for its energizing and invigorating effects. Practitioners often report heightened mental clarity and focus, making it especially beneficial as a morning practice or as preparation for meditation.

However, it's essential to approach Kapalabhati with caution. Since it involves forceful breathing, it is generally recommended for experienced practitioners and is contraindicated for those with high blood pressure, heart conditions, or respiratory issues. Beginners should start slowly, focusing on proper technique rather than speed, and always practice on an empty stomach.

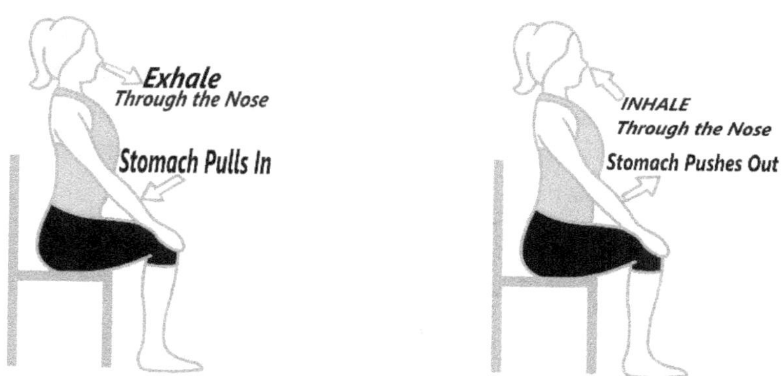

2. Yoga

- Restorative Yoga Poses: Gentle yoga poses like Child's Pose, Cat-Cow, and Legs-Up-The-Wall pose. These poses encourage relaxation and deep breathing, which stimulates the vagus nerve.

- Pranayama Practices: Breathing techniques in yoga, such as Nadi Shodhana (alternate nostril breathing), can enhance vagal tone by promoting relaxation and balanced breathing.

3. Meditation and Mindfulness Practices

- Guided Meditation: Focuses on deep relaxation and stress reduction, contributing to parasympathetic activation.

- Mindfulness Meditation: Encourages present-moment awareness and calmness, stimulating the vagus nerve.

4. Tai Chi and Qigong

- These traditional Chinese exercises combine slow, deliberate movements with deep breathing, promoting relaxation and enhancing vagal function.

5. Aerobic Exercises

- Moderate Intensity Cardiovascular Exercise: Activities like brisk walking, light jogging, or swimming, performed moderately, can improve heart rate variability, indicating better vagal tone.

6. Singing, Humming, and Gargling

- The vagus nerve, which is associated with the vocal cords and muscles in the back of the throat, receives mechanical stimulation from these activities.

6.a *The OM Sound*

The Om (or Aum) sound is usually pronounced as a long "AUM" or "OM", with three distinct phases:

1. It begins with an "Aah" sound (like in "father"), starting from the back of the throat.

2. This transitions into an "Oo" sound (like in "who"), with the lips forming a circle.

3. Finally, it ends with an "Mm" sound, with the lips closed, creating a vibration that can be felt in the sinuses and skull.

The entire sound is typically elongated and can last several seconds. It often starts at a higher pitch and gradually lowers, with the "Mm" portion usually being the lowest and potentially trailing off into silence.

6.b *Correlation between the Om sound of meditation and the vagus nerve.*

There's an interesting potential connection between the "Om" sound used in meditation and the vagus nerve. Here's a brief overview:

1. *Om Sound*:

- A sacred syllable in various Eastern religions, often used in meditation practices.

- Typically chanted at a low frequency.

2. *Vagus nerve*:

- The longest cranial nerve, connecting the brain to various organs.

- Plays a crucial role in the parasympathetic nervous system, which promotes relaxation.

3. *Potential correlation*:

- Low-frequency sounds, like the Om chant, may stimulate the vagus nerve.

- This stimulation could activate the parasympathetic response, leading to relaxation.

4. *Possible mechanisms*:

- Vibrations from the chant may physically stimulate the nerve.

- The act of chanting itself involves controlled breathing, which can affect vagal tone.

5. *Potential benefits*:

- Reduced stress and anxiety

- Lowered heart rate and blood pressure

- Improved mood and focus

While there's some scientific interest in this connection, more research is needed to fully understand the relationship between Om chanting and vagus nerve stimulation.

6.c *Let's delve deeper into some key aspects of this potential correlation:*

1. *The science behind Om chanting*:

Om chanting typically produces a fundamental frequency around 130-140 Hz, with harmonics extending into higher frequencies. This low-frequency vibration is believed to resonate throughout the body, potentially affecting various physiological systems.

2. *Vagus Nerve Stimulation (VNS)*:

The vagus nerve is sensitive to both mechanical and electrical stimulation. Traditional VNS involves surgically implanted devices, but researchers are exploring non-invasive methods, including sound-based stimulation.

3. *Respiratory Sinus Arrhythmia (RSA)*:

Chanting Om involves slow, controlled breathing, which can enhance RSA - the natural variation in heart rate that occurs during the breathing cycle. Strong RSA is associated with higher vagal tone and better autonomic nervous system function.

4. *Neuroimaging Studies*:

Some studies have shown that Om chanting activates areas of the brain associated with vagus nerve function, such as the orbitofrontal and anterior cingulate cortices, insula, and thalamus.

5. *Potential therapeutic applications*:

Researchers are investigating whether practices like Om chanting could be used as a complementary therapy for conditions associated with low vagal tone, such as depression, anxiety, and inflammatory disorders.

6. *Broader context of sound therapy*:

The potential Om-vagus nerve connection fits into a wider field of research on how different sound frequencies might affect human physiology, including studies on binaural beats and other forms of sound healing.

7. *Challenges in research*:

Studying this connection is complex due to the subjective nature of meditation experiences and the difficulty in isolating the specific effects of the Om sound from other aspects of meditative practices.

6.d *Vibrational Meditations*

Vibrational meditations can effectively stimulate the vagus nerve through sound. Humming or singing are common methods, and Bhuta recommends chanting "om" or a longer mantra such as "om mani padme hum" during meditation. Additionally, ujjayi breath, often referred to as

Darth Vader breath, involves creating a deep throat sound during breathing and is frequently practiced in yoga, which also aids in vagal stimulation through breath and movement.

Another technique, Bhramari pranayama or buzzing breath, involves placing four fingers over your eyes and closing your ears with your thumbs. You inhale deeply through your nose, close your eyes, and exhale while making a humming sound with your lips closed.

"Sound-based breathing creates a buzzing sensation in the brain, which can help drown out stress and intrusive thoughts, leading to relaxation," Bhuta explains.

No matter which meditation you choose, it will help you remain balanced and composed. Bhuta notes that many people are stuck in a constant state of fight-or-flight, driven by adrenaline, which disrupts the functions controlled by the vagus nerve. Taking time to slow down and enter a restful state periodically helps maintain a calm nervous system.

7. Laughter Yoga

- Laughter naturally stimulates deep diaphragmatic breathing and is a powerful activator of the parasympathetic nervous system. Laughter Yoga is practiced as a remedy for physical, psychological, and spiritual well-being, based on the belief that intentional (simulated) laughter offers the same benefits as spontaneous laughter, such as laughing at a joke

8. Cold Exposure

- Short cold showers or cold-water splashes on the face can activate the vagus nerve. It initially causes a slight stress response, followed by a significant parasympathetic rebound. Applying something cold behind the neck can slow the heart rate and increase activation of the vagal nerve, or you can adopt a careful cryotherapy treatment in an ice bath with Cold Water Immersion (5-15 minutes).

9. Progressive Muscle Relaxation

- It involves tension and relaxation in sequence of different muscle groups, which can help in reducing physical tension and triggering the relaxation response of the vagus nerve.

10. Reflexology and Massage

- A targeted massage, especially in the area of the neck, head and feet, can stimulate the vagus nerve, favoring relaxation and reducing stress.

10.a. Emotional Freedom Technique (EFT)

How to Tap Your Anxiety Away With Tapping Meditation

Emotional Freedom Technique (EFT) Tapping is a holistic acupressure treatment that can help alleviate conditions like PTSD, overeating, and depression. This technique involves tapping on specific points on the body while focusing on emotional distress, helping to regulate the body's stress response.

What Is Emotional Freedom Tapping?

EFT Tapping involves using your fingertips to gently tap on specific points on the body, corresponding to traditional Chinese medicine acupressure points. According to Nick Ortner, CEO of The Tapping Solution, this sends calming signals to the brain, letting it know it's safe to relax, thus turning off the fight-or-flight response.

Benefits of EFT

Research supports the benefits of EFT. A 2020 study in *Psychological Trauma* showed that participants practicing EFT experienced a 50% decrease in anxiety and a 43% decrease in cortisol levels. EFT can help with:

- Anxiety and depression

- PTSD

- Phobias

- Weight loss

- Sleep problems

- Physical pain

How to Practice EFT

1. **Identify an Issue**: Focus on something bothering you, like fear, anxiety, or a physical ailment.

2. **Rate the Intensity**: On a scale from 0 to 10, rate the issue's intensity.

3. **Create a Setup Statement**: Acknowledge your distress while accepting yourself. For example, "Even though I have this [problem], I deeply and completely accept myself."

4. **Tap on the Points**: Tap on nine major points along the body's meridians while maintaining mental focus on the issue.

5. **Reassess the Intensity**: Rate the intensity again to see if there's a change.

But, which are the 12 primary meridians in the body, their functions, symptoms of imbalance, and how to rebalance them using EFT (Emotional Freedom Techniques) tapping points?

Each meridian is associated with a specific organ, emotion, and time of day when its energy is most active. When a meridian is imbalanced, it can lead to physical, emotional, and mental health issues. By understanding these meridians and their optimal energy flow times, one can use targeted energy exercises and EFT tapping to promote better health. Here's a brief overview of the meridians:

Meridian	Function	Associated Emotion	Active Time
1.Lung Meridian	Regulates breathing	Grief	3:00 – 5:00 AM
2. Large Intestine Meridian	Processes waste	Letting go	5:00 – 7:00 AM
3. Stomach Meridian	Digests food	Worry	7:00 – 9:00 AM
4. Spleen Meridian	Distributes nutrients	Fatigue	9:00 – 11:00 AM
5.Heart Meridian	Circulates blood	Joy	11:00 – 1:00 PM
6.Small Intestine Meridian	Distributes nutrients	—	1:00 – 3:00 PM
7. Bladder Meridian	Removes waste	Anger	3:00 – 5:00 PM
8. Kidney Meridian	Regulates reproduction, willpower	—	5:00 – 7:00 PM
9. Pericardium Meridian	Protects the heart	Emotional balance	7:00 – 9:00 PM
10. Triple Warmer Meridian	Regulates metabolism, stress	—	9:00 – 11:00 PM
11. Gallbladder Meridian	Expels bile, supports decision-making	—	11:00 – 1:00 AM
12. Liver Meridian	Circulates energy	Anger	1:00 – 3:00 AM

Here there are the **_9 Tapping Points_** used in EFT and the meridian lines they correspond to:

- **Top of the Head (TH)** - Governing & Bladder Meridian -

  Location: Top and center of the head

- **Inner Eyebrow (EB)** - Bladder & Stomach Meridian –

  Location: Above the nose, where the eyebrow starts on each side.

- **Side of Eye (SE)** - Gallbladder, Triple Warmer, & Small Intestine Meridian-

  Location: The bone on the outside corner of each eye.

- **Under Eye (UE)** - Stomach Meridian –

  Location: An inch below the pupil on the bone beneath each eye.

- **Under Nose (UN)** - Governing Vessel & Large Intestine Meridian-

  Location: Between the bottom of the nose and the top of the upper lip.

- **Chin Point (CH)** - Conception Vessel (Central Meridian) & Stomach Meridian –

  Location: Between the chin and lower lip.

- **Inner Collarbone (CB)** - Kidney Meridian –

  Location: Below each collarbone, an inch to the left or right of the center of the body.

- **Under Arm (UA)** - Spleen Meridian –

  Location: Four inches below the armpit on each side of the body.

- **Karate Chop (KC)**- Bladder Meridian -

  Location: The side of each hand, between the pinky finger and the wrist.

Each meridian has a corresponding EFT tapping point, allowing for emotional and physical energy balancing through tapping exercises.

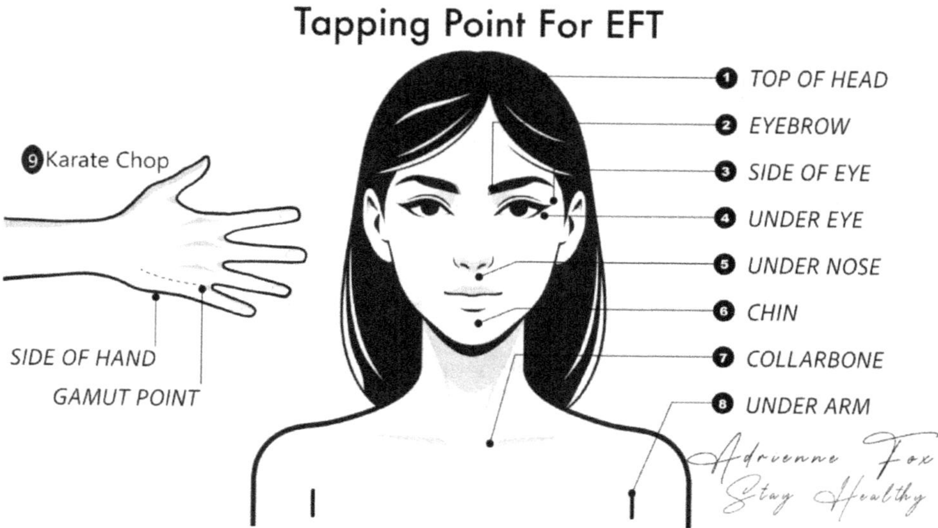

Finding a Practitioner

While EFT can be practiced alone, working with a practitioner can be beneficial. They provide a safe space to explore emotions, help identify core issues and formulate effective tapping statements. Look for consultations and local EFT workshops to find a practitioner you feel comfortable with.

EFT can be a valuable addition to your mental health toolkit, offering a non-invasive, gentle method to reduce stress and improve overall well-being. Always consult with a healthcare provider for severe mental health concerns and consider combining EFT with traditional treatment.

6.3: Integrating Vagal Exercises into Daily Routines

Creating a balanced exercise regime tailored to improve vagal tone involves incorporating a variety of exercises that stimulate the parasympathetic nervous system and enhance overall well-being. Your goal is to structure a routine that blends cardiovascular, strength, flexibility, and relaxation exercises throughout the week. Here's a guide on how to create such a routine, considering different fitness levels and preferences:

Weekly Exercise Plan for Vagal Tone Enhancement

> ***Day 1: Cardiovascular Exercise***

- Activity: Moderate Intensity Cardio (e.g., brisk walking, light jogging, cycling, or swimming)

- Duration: 30-45 minutes

- Focus: Enhance heart rate variability and improve blood circulation.

- Adaptation for Beginners: Start with low-impact activities like brisk walking or stationary cycling for 20-30 minutes.

> ***Day 2: Strength Training***

- Activity: Strength training for the whole body, with particular attention to the main muscle groups.

- Duration: 30-45 minutes

- Focus: Build muscle strength and resilience, regulate stress hormones.

- Adaptation for Beginners: Use lighter weights or bodyweight exercises; focus on form and controlled movements.

✓ ***Day 3: Yoga or Pilates***

- Activity: A yoga session focusing on relaxation poses or a Pilates class

- Duration: 30-60 minutes

- Focus: Stimulate the vagus nerve through deep breathing and mindful movements.

- Adaptation for Beginners: Choose gentle yoga styles like Hatha or Yin Yoga, or beginner-friendly Pilates classes.

> ➤ ***Day 4: Active Recovery***

- Activity: Light activity like leisurely walking, easy cycling, or restorative yoga

- Duration: 20-30 minutes

- Focus: Active recovery to reduce muscle soreness and hold mobility.

- Adaptation for All Levels: Adjust the intensity to ensure it's relaxing and rejuvenating.

> ✓ ***Day 5: Flexibility and Mobility Work***

- Activity: Stretching routine or a mobility-focused exercise session

- Duration: 20-30 minutes

- Focus: Improve flexibility, reduce muscle tension, and enhance parasympathetic activation.

- Adaptation for All Levels: Tailor the stretching to individual flexibility levels; use props if needed.

> ✓ ***Day 6: High-Intensity Interval Training (HIIT) – Optional***

- Activity: HIIT session

- Duration: 20-30 minutes

- Focus: Improve cardiovascular health and metabolism.

- Adaptation for Beginners: Lower the intensity and duration; incorporate more rest periods.

➢ *Day 7: Mindfulness and Relaxation Exercises*

- Activity: Guided meditation, deep breathing exercises, or laughter yoga

- Duration: 20-30 minutes

- Focus: Directly stimulate the vagus nerve to enhance relaxation and stress management.

- Adaptation for All Levels: Choose activities that are enjoyable and calming, and suitable for all fitness levels.

❑ *General Tips for Optimizing the Routine*

1. Personalization: Tailor the routine to individual preferences and fitness levels. Always start at a comfortable level and progressively enhance intensity.

2. Consistency: Regularity is key in any exercise regime. Encourage sticking to the routine for long-term benefits.

3. Listening to the Body: Educate about the importance of regulating the body's signals. Modify the routine if any exercise causes discomfort.

4. Combining Exercises: For those with time constraints, combine activities, like strength training with yoga or Pilates.

5. Monitoring Progress: Keep track of improvements in overall well-being, stress levels, and physical fitness.

7.1 Sleep Hygiene for Vagal Health

7.1.a <u>Understanding the Connection Between Sleep and the Vagus Nerve</u>

- *Physiological Role of Sleep*: Sleep is fundamental to our overall health, and it plays a critical role in the functioning of the vagus nerve. During restful sleep, the body activates its parasympathetic nervous system, which is largely mediated by the vagus nerve. This restorative state is essential for balancing bodily functions regulated by the vagus nerve, including heart rate and digestion.

- *Impact of Poor Sleep on Vagal Tone*: Lack of quality sleep can lead to decreased vagal tone, manifesting in symptoms like increased stress levels, poor digestion, and imbalances in heart rate variability (HRV). Chronic sleep deprivation can exacerbate these issues, leading to a cycle of stress and poor vagal function.

7.1.b <u>Principles of Sleep Hygiene for Enhancing Vagal Health</u>

- *Consistent Sleep Schedule*: Regular hours of sleep and wakefulness help to regulate the body's internal clock, promoting better quality sleep and vagal health.

- *Optimal Sleep Environment*: Creating a sleep-conducive environment – cool, dark, and quiet – can considerably advance sleep quality. The use of comfortable bedding and minimizing light and noise pollution are key factors.

- *Pre-Sleep Routine*: Establishing a calming pre-sleep routine, such as reading, light stretching, or listening to soft music, can promote relaxation and prepare the body for sleep.

7.1.c Diet and Sleep

- *Nutritional Considerations*: Dietary choices can impact sleep quality.

In healthy eating, before bedtime, it is best to avoid drinks, such as coffee and alcohol, and heavy foods or meals. Conversely, for better sleep, it's best to favor foods and drinks that contain tryptophan or magnesium.

7.1.d Managing Evening Stress

- Relaxation Before Bedtime: Techniques to reduce stress before bedtime are crucial. This can include mindfulness practices, deep breathing exercises, or journaling, all of which can calm the mind and enhance the body's readiness for sleep.

7.2 Relaxation Techniques That Work

7.2.a Integrating Relaxation into Daily Life

- *Importance of Regular Relaxation*: Regular relaxation is essential for maintaining a healthy vagal tone.

7.2.b Breathing Techniques for Relaxation

- *Focused Breathing Exercises*: Techniques like diaphragmatic breathing, box breathing, and guided breathing exercises are effective for immediate stress relief and can be practiced almost anywhere, anytime.

7.2.c Mindfulness and Meditation

- *Meditation Practices*: Various forms of meditation, including guided meditation, mindfulness meditation, and loving-kindness meditation, are discussed for their benefits in reducing stress and enhancing vagal tone.

- *Mindfulness in Daily Activities*: A simple yet powerful way to promote relaxation is to integrate mindfulness into everyday activities, such as eating or walking.

About Chakra & Vagus Nerve

"Chakra" is a term originating from ancient Indian philosophy and spiritual practices, particularly within the traditions of Hinduism and Buddhism. The word "chakra" in Sanskrit, an ancient Indian language, literally means "wheel" or "disk." In the context of spiritual and energy practices, chakras are conceptualized as centers of energy within the human body.

According to these traditions Chakras are vital energy centers that lie along the spine, starting from the base to the top of the head. Each chakra is thought to correspond to specific organs, nerves, and aspects of our emotional, physical, and spiritual well-being. There are traditionally seven main chakras, and each is correlated with a specific color, element, and set of characteristics:

1. *Root Chakra* (Muladhara): Positioned at the base of the spine, it is linked with **red** and represents grounding, stability, and basic needs.

2. *Sacral Chakra* (Svadhishthana): Situated in the lower abdomen, it is linked with **orange** and represents creativity, sexuality, and emotional balance.

3. *Solar Plexus Chakra* (Manipura): Identified in the top abdomen, with color **yellow,** and represents personal power, self-confidence, and self-control.

4. *Heart Chakra* (Anahata): Found in the center of the chest, it is linked with **green** and symbolizes love, compassion, and acceptance.

5. *Throat Chakra* (Vishuddha): Located in the throat, it is related with **blue** and represents communication, expression, and truth.

6. *Third Eye Chakra* (Ajna): Situated on the forehead between the eyes, it is linked with the color **indigo** and represents intuition, imagination, and wisdom.

7. *Crown Chakra* (Sahasrara): At the top of the head, with **violet or white**, represents spiritual connection and enlightenment.

(Download the descriptive images found at the end of the book !!)

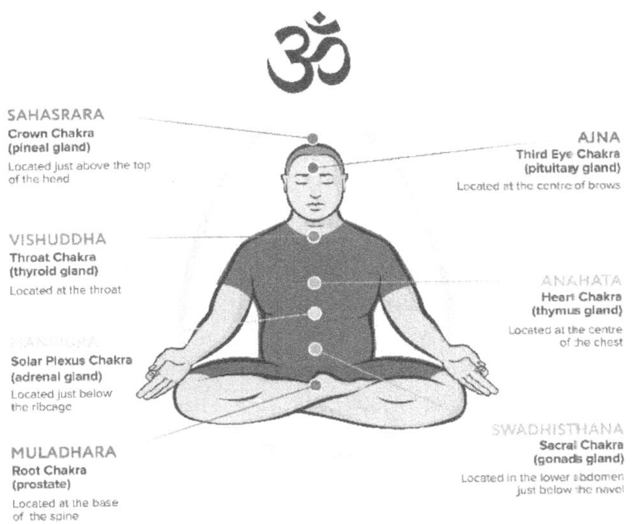

Chakras of human body
Ayurveda, Yoga, Buddhism and Hinduism
ADREINNE FOX -STAY HEALTHY

In various spiritual and healing practices, maintaining the balance and alignment of these chakras is considered essential for physical, emotional, and spiritual health.

The connection between the chakras and the vagus nerve is an area of interest that blends concepts from traditional Eastern spiritual practices with Western physiological understanding. In Eastern cultures, the chakras are regarded as energy centers that are present throughout the body, and each one represents a distinct aspect of physical, emotional, and spiritual well-being.

While traditional Western medicine does not typically incorporate the concept of chakras, there is growing interest in how the vagus nerve's function might intersect with what chakras represent in terms of energy flow and balance. Various exercises and modalities that are thought to stimulate the vagus nerve may also be seen as influencing the chakras. Here are some examples:

1. *Meditation and Mindfulness:* Practices like meditation and mindfulness can stimulate the vagus nerve, promoting relaxation and

stress reduction. These practices are also seen as beneficial for balancing the chakras, particularly the third eye (Ajna) and crown (Sahasrara) chakras, which are associated with intuition and higher consciousness.

2. *Yoga*: Many yoga poses are evaluated to activate and balance different chakras. For instance, heart-opening poses like backbends may stimulate the heart chakra (Anahata), while poses like forward bends can stimulate the root chakra (Muladhara). Yoga also stimulates the vagus nerve, particularly through controlled breathing (pranayama) and relaxation techniques.

3. *Breathing Exercises* (Pranayama): Breathing techniques, especially those that emphasize slow and deep breathing, activate the vagus nerve, which helps regulate the heart rate and induce a state of calm. These exercises are also integral to yoga and are thought to help balance the chakras.

4. *Chanting and Singing*: Chanting, singing, and even humming can stimulate the vagus nerve due to the vibration of the vocal cords. This is also seen in practices like mantra chanting, which is believed to activate the throat chakra (Vishuddha), associated with communication and self-expression.

5. *Aromatherapy*: Certain scents are believed to help in balancing specific chakras. For example, lavender can be calming and is often associated with the third eye chakra. Aromatherapy has the ability to calm the vagus nerve as well.

6. *Reiki and Energy Healing*: These practices focus on the transfer and balancing of energy, often directly related to the chakras. While more research is needed, some suggest that such energy work can influence the body's physiological processes, potentially impacting the vagus nerve.

7. *Diet and Nutrition*: Certain foods are thought to correspond with chakra health. For example, root vegetables are often associated with the root chakra, and green leafy vegetables with the heart chakra. A balanced diet also supports the overall function of the vagus nerve.

- Yoga and Stretching:

Gentle yoga and stretching can release muscle tension and facilitate a state of rest. **Example:**

Cat&Cow Stretch

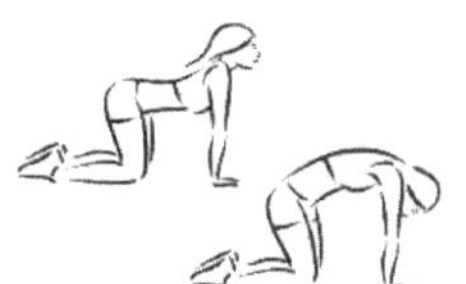

Inhale and tilt the pelvis for cow laying, exhalation and insert the tailbone for cat laying.

Child Pose Stretch

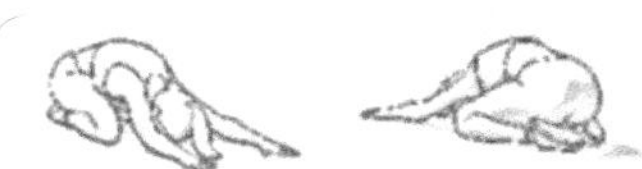

Spread your knees as wide as the mattress. Leave your belly between your thighs and place your forehead on the floor.

Cobra Pose Stretch

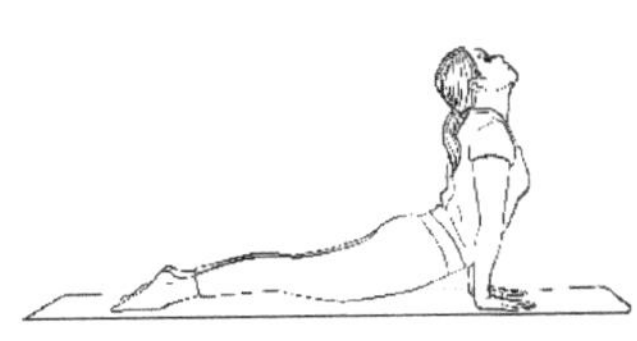

Make sure your pelvis and legs are firmly anchored to the floor while you lift your chest.

Wall Pose

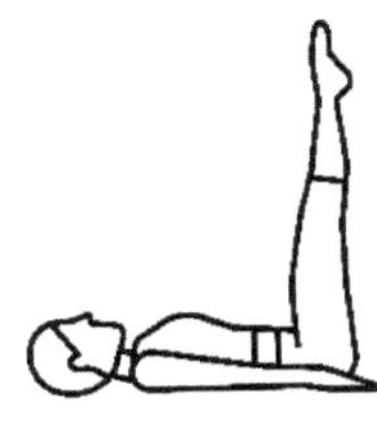

Sit on the floor in front of a wall. Lower your shoulders and head towards the floor. Adjust the position by moving the tailbone towards the wall and lift and stretch the legs along the wall.

7.2.e <u>Leveraging Technology for Relaxation</u>

- *Apps and Online Resources*: The technology world now offers many apps and smartwatches to perform meditation and breathing techniques, with sounds, music, and explanations. We invite you to explore and consult these new resources.

7.2.f <u>Building a Personal Relaxation Routine</u>

- *Customizing Relaxation Techniques*: it is recommended to customize and combine different relaxation techniques to create a personal routine that resonates with individual preferences and schedules. It is crucial to discover what works best for each individual and to make relaxation a regular part of one's life.

7.2.d <u>Physical Relaxation Techniques</u>

- *Progressive Muscle Relaxation (PMR)*: A step-by-step guide to practicing PMR, a method that involves tensing and relaxing different muscle groups, is provided. This technique is particularly effective in reducing physical tension and promoting a sense of calm.

How it works

As you breathe in, tense a specific group of muscles (like your upper thighs) for 5 to 10 seconds, then exhale and quickly let go of the tension in those muscles.

Allow yourself a relaxation period of 10 to 20 seconds before moving to the next group of muscles (such as your buttocks).

When you relieve the tension, concentrate on the sensations you experience as the muscles relax.

Using imagery can enhance this process; envision that stress is leaving your body with each muscle group you relax.

Progressively move up your body, alternating between tensing and calming several muscle groups.

8.1 Understanding Vagus Nerve Stimulation (VNS)

8.1.a <u>Overview of Vagus Nerve Stimulation</u>

- *Introduction to VNS*:

Vagus Nerve Stimulation is a unique therapeutic approach that targets the vagus nerve, one of the longest cranial nerves in the body.

VNS involves the use of a device that generates electrical impulses. These impulses are delivered to the vagus nerve, typically via a surgically implanted device, with the aim of modulating the nerve's activity.

The history of VNS is both fascinating and rich in medical innovation. The concept of VNS emerged from the understanding that electrical stimulation of the nervous system could yield therapeutic benefits. Initially, VNS was developed as a treatment for epilepsy, a neurological condition characterized by recurrent seizures. The rationale behind using VNS for epilepsy stemmed from the observation that stimulating the vagus nerve could influence brain activity and potentially reduce the frequency and intensity of seizures.

In its early stages, VNS showed promising results in managing epilepsy, specifically in circumstances where traditional medications were ineffective. This success paved the way for further research and development, leading to the refinement of VNS devices and techniques. The initial use of VNS in epilepsy treatment was a significant milestone, as it opened new avenues for exploring the therapeutic potential of nerve stimulation.

- *Mechanism of VNS*:

The topic "Mechanism of VNS" delves into the intricate workings of Vagus Nerve Stimulation (VNS), a sophisticated medical therapy used primarily for treating conditions like epilepsy. At the heart of VNS is a small device, often likened to a pacemaker, which is surgically implanted under the skin. This device is the key to the therapy's effectiveness, as it is responsible for delivering regular, mild pulses of electrical energy directly to the vagus nerve.

The vagus nerve extends from the brainstem to various organs. When this nerve is electrically stimulated through the VNS device, it influences the nerve's activity and, consequently, the various bodily functions it controls.

One of the primary applications of VNS is in the management of epilepsy, a neurological disorder characterized by recurrent seizures. These are essentially episodes of abnormal electrical activity in the brain. The electrical impulses delivered by the VNS device to the vagus nerve can help establish this abnormal brain activity. By modulating the nerve's activity, VNS can bring a level of stability to the brain's electrical environment.

The efficiency of VNS in reducing the frequency of seizures in epilepsy patients has been a significant breakthrough. VNS offers a viable alternative for many patients, principally for those who do not respond well to conventional epilepsy medications. The electrical stimulation provided by the VNS device is typically mild but consistent, ensuring that the vagus nerve is continually influenced to maintain a more stable electrical state in the brain.

8.1.b Expanding Applications of VNS

- *VNS for Depression*: The application of VNS has expanded beyond epilepsy; in fact, it is used in the treatment of major depressive disorders, especially in cases where patients have not responded to conventional treatments.

- *VNS in Other Conditions*: Recent research is exploring the potential of VNS for other conditions, such as anxiety disorders, chronic pain, and heart disease.

8.1.c <u>Benefits and Risks of VNS</u>

- *Efficacy and Advantages*: The benefits of VNS are in the ability to provide long-term relief from the first symptoms and improve quality of life, are outlined.

- *Potential Side Effects and Considerations*: VNS, while beneficial for many, is not without its drawbacks, and understanding these is essential for making an informed decision.

VNS implies the surgical implantation of a device that delivers electrical impulses to the vagus nerve. While this procedure has shown effectiveness in treating conditions like epilepsy and depression, it can also lead to certain side effects. Commonly reported side effects include hoarseness or changes in voice tone, which occur due to the proximity of the vagus nerve to the voice box. Patients may notice a distinct change in their voice quality, especially when the device is actively delivering electrical pulses.

Throat pain or discomfort is another side effect that some patients experience. The range of this can be between mild and moderate and is usually related to the stimulation of the vagus nerve. In some cases, individuals may also experience shortness of breath or breathing difficulties. This is again attributable to the nerve's role in regulating respiratory functions.

It is important for individuals considering VNS to understand these potential side effects and weigh them against the benefits of the procedure. While many patients experience significant improvements in their conditions, the decision to undergo VNS must be taken after a thorough discussion with healthcare professionals. This includes a comprehensive evaluation of the individual's medical history, recent health status, and the seriousness of their condition.

Additionally, patients should be aware that the side effects of VNS can vary in intensity and may change over time. Some side effects may diminish as the body adjusts to the device, while others might persist.

Continuous communication with health professionals is critical to effectively managing side effects.

8.2.a <u>Recognizing the Need for Professional Intervention</u>

- *Identifying Symptoms*: Understanding when to seek professional help is a vital step in managing one's health. Often, individuals may try to manage symptoms on their own or delay seeking help due to various reasons, including uncertainty about the severity of their condition. Let's try to understate these ambiguities, to encourage timely professional consultation.

In the realm of mental health, symptoms that necessitate professional intervention include enduring feelings of sadness, hopelessness, anxiety, or thoughts of self-harm. If these symptoms are severe, unrelenting, and interfere with daily functioning, it is crucial to seek help from a mental health professional. Mental health disorders, such as major depressive disorder, generalized anxiety disorder, or other mood disorders, can significantly impact quality of life, but they are treatable with the right professional guidance.

Chronic pain is another area where professional intervention is often necessary. If pain persists despite standard treatments and home remedies, or if it begins to affect mobility, sleep, or quality of life, consulting a healthcare provider is essential. Chronic pain can be a symptom of various underlying conditions and requires a thorough evaluation to determine the appropriate treatment.

Intractable epilepsy, characterized by seizures that are resistant to medication, is a particularly critical condition where professional intervention is imperative. Uncontrolled seizures can pose significant risks and impact an individual's safety and well-being. Neurologists or epilepsy specialists can offer advanced treatment options, including medication adjustments, surgical interventions, or therapies like Vagus Nerve Stimulation (VNS).

One needs to be vigilant about one's symptoms, assessing and understanding whether it is necessary to seek help from professionals, as a sign of strength and not weakness. Early intervention can lead to better therapeutic outcomes, improved quality of life, and in some cases, can be lifesaving.

It is important to recognize the limitation of self-managed care, especially when dealing with serious conditions that could potentially benefit from therapies.

8.2.b <u>Consultation and Evaluation Process</u>

- *Seeking a Specialist*: The first step in this process is identifying the right specialist. For VNS and similar therapies, this typically involves neurologists, neurosurgeons, or psychiatrists who have specific training and experience in administering these treatments. Finding a specialist with a robust background in the specific condition being treated is essential. This can be done through referrals from primary care physicians, recommendations from patient advocacy groups, or by researching medical centers and hospitals that have a strong neurology or psychiatry department.

Once a potential specialist is identified, preparing for the consultation is the next critical step. This preparation involves gathering all relevant medical records, including previous treatment histories, medication lists, and any diagnostic test results. It's also important to prepare a list of symptoms, recording their frequency, severity, and any triggers or alleviating factors. This information provides the specialist with a comprehensive view of the patient's clinical history and current condition.

Patients should also prepare a list of questions for the specialist. These might include inquiries about the specialist's experience with VNS or other advanced therapies, the risks and benefits of the treatment, what the procedure entails, recovery time, and what outcomes can be expected. Understanding the financial factors such as insurance coverage and costs, is also crucial.

During the consultation, the specialist will assess the patient's suitability for VNS or other therapies. This evaluation may involve a detailed medical examination, a revision of the patient's medical history, and possibly additional diagnostic tests. The specialist will discuss the potential benefits and risks of the treatment, what the procedure involves, and what the patient can expect in terms of recovery and long-term management.

The consultation and evaluation process are a collaborative endeavor between the patient and the specialist. It is an opportunity for patients to gain a thorough understanding of their treatment options and for specialists to develop a tailored treatment plan that aligns with the patient's specific needs and health goals.

8.2.c <u>Understanding the Journey of Advanced Therapies</u>

- *Setting Expectations*: Advanced therapies, particularly those like VNS, involve a multifaceted journey that extends beyond the actual medical procedure. One of the key phases discussed in this section is the typical timeline of such therapies. This includes the pre-treatment evaluation, the scheduling and execution of the procedure, the recovery period, and the long-term management of the therapy. For instance, in the case of VNS, the timeline might encompass initial consultations, the surgical implantation of the device, post-operative recovery, and regular follow-ups for device adjustments.

Advanced therapies like VNS are not one-time solutions but rather part of a continuous treatment strategy. This might involve regular visits to the healthcare provider for device check-ups and adjustments, monitoring for any side effects or complications, and assessing the therapy's effectiveness over time. Patients may need to be patient and persistent, as the full benefits of such treatments might only become apparent after an extended period.

Another crucial aspect covered is setting realistic expectations about outcomes. While advanced therapies can offer significant improvements in conditions like epilepsy or severe depression, they may not be a cure. Patients might experience a reduction in symptoms or an improved quality of life, but it is important to have a realistic understanding of what these treatments can and cannot achieve.

It is important to keep an open line of communication with healthcare providers as a vital part of this path. Patients are encouraged to actively engage with their doctors, ask questions, express concerns, and report any changes in their condition. This ongoing dialogue is essential for the effective management of the therapy and for making any necessary adjustments to the treatment plan.

- *Support and Follow-up Care*: Post-procedure care is multifaceted and begins immediately after the patient has undergone the treatment. One of the key components of this care is regular check-ups. These check-ups are essential for monitoring the patient's progress, assessing the effectiveness of the treatment, and ensuring that the patient is recovering as expected. For treatments like VNS, these check-ups may involve evaluating the device's functionality, checking for any physical complications, and discussing any changes in the patient's symptoms or overall health.

Device adjustments are often a necessary part of follow-up care, especially in treatments involving implantable devices like in VNS. Over time, the patient's condition may change, or the initial settings of the device may need fine-tuning to achieve optimal results. Regular follow-up appointments give healthcare professionals the opportunity to make these adjustments. This could involve changing the intensity, frequency, or duration of the electrical impulses in the case of VNS, ensuring that the patient receives the most therapeutic benefit from the treatment.

Managing side effects is a crucial aspect of care and follow-up. Although advanced therapies can offer significant benefits, they can also involve side effects. Patients need to be prepared for this possibility and have strategies in place for dealing with any adverse effects that arise. This could include medication to manage symptoms, lifestyle changes to mitigate side effects, or additional therapies to complement the primary treatment.

The role of support systems in this process cannot be overstated. The support of family, friends, and support groups can be invaluable for patients navigating the recovery and adjustment period following advanced therapies. Emotional and practical support can help patients cope with the changes in their health and lifestyle that may accompany such treatments.

Customizable Vagus Nerve Health Plans for Different Lifestyles

Lifestyle Category	Key Focus Areas	Suggested Activities	Notes
Busy Professionals	Stress Management, Efficient Exercise, Quick Healthy Meals	- 10-min guided meditation during breaks- 30-min HIIT sessions 3 times a week- Meal prep with anti-inflammatory foods	Prioritize activities that fit into a busy schedule
Parents	Stress Reduction, Family Activities, Simple Nutrition	- Family yoga sessions on weekends- Healthy meal planning with kids- Short breathing exercises during the day	Include family-friendly and time-efficient activities
Students	Balanced Diet, Regular Exercise, Stress Management	Study breaks with stretching or short walks- Cafeteria choices rich in probiotics- Weekly group sports or fitness classes	Focus on integrating health habits into study routine
Retirees	Gentle Physical Activity, Social Engagement, Relaxation	Daily walks or light gardening- Joining social clubs or groups- Regular practice of mindfulness or tai chi	Emphasize activities that enhance social interaction and mobility

Monitoring progress and adaptation of the vagus nerve health approach

Goal/Aspect	Method of Tracking	Frequency of Evaluation	Adjustment Strategy
Stress Reduction	Journaling stress levels<>Use of apps for meditation adherence	Bi-weekly	Try different relaxation techniques if current ones are ineffective
Sleep Quality	Sleep tracking apps<>Sleep diary	Monthly	Adjust sleep environment or routine if quality doesn't improve
Diet Changes	Food diary<>Weekly meal planning review	Weekly	Introduce new recipes or foods if monotony sets in
Exercise Routine	Fitness tracker data<>Exercise log	Weekly	Change workout types or intensities if goals are not being met
Overall Well-being	Self-assessment questionnaires <>Regular health check-ups	Monthly	Consult health professionals for personalized advice if needed

These case studies, in a tabular format, represent various backgrounds and their successful journey in improving vagal health. Each case includes background information, the strategies used for transformation, the impact of these changes, and the long-term implications for health and lifestyle.

Table 1: Diverse Backgrounds, Common Goal

Case Study	Background	Vagal Health Issue	Goal
Case 1: Alex	30-year-old software developer	Chronic stress, anxiety	Reduce stress, improve mental clarity
Case 2: Maria	45-year-old schoolteacher	Poor digestion, irregular heartbeat	Enhance digestive health, stabilize heart rate
Case 3: David	55-year-old retired veteran	Insomnia, mood swings	Improve sleep quality, emotional balance
Case 4: Emma	38-year-old stay-at-home parent	Postpartum depression, fatigue	Alleviate depression symptoms, increase energy levels

Table 2: Strategies and Transformations

Case Study	Strategies Used	Transformations Observed
Case 1: Alex	Mindfulness meditation, yoga, dietary changes (increased omega-3s)	Reduced anxiety levels, better focus on work
Case 2: Maria	Probiotic-rich diet, regular walking, deep breathing exercises	Improved digestion, more regular heart rate
Case 3: David	Tai chi, sleep hygiene practices, vagus nerve stimulation therapy	Enhanced sleep quality, more stable mood
Case 4: Emma	Aerobic exercise, joining a support group, guided relaxation techniques	Decreased depressive symptoms, more daily energy

Table 3: Understanding the Impact

Case Study	Physical Health Benefits	Mental/Emotional Benefits
Case 1: Alex	Lower blood pressure, improved HRV	Greater stress resilience, enhanced cognitive function
Case 2: Maria	Better gut health, stabilized cardiovascular function	Increased overall well-being, reduced stress
Case 3: David	Improved sleep patterns, better autonomic balance	Emotional stability, reduced symptoms of depression
Case 4: Emma	Increased physical stamina, better immune response	Elevated mood, improved coping skills

Table 4: Long-term Health and Lifestyle Implications

Case Study	Lifestyle Changes	Long-term Health Outlook
Case 1: Alex	Integrated meditation into daily routine, healthier eating habits	Sustainable stress management, reduced risk of chronic stress-related health issues
Case 2: Maria	Regular physical activity, mindful eating	Ongoing digestive health, maintained heart health
Case 3: David	Consistent sleep schedule, continued practice of tai chi	Long-term emotional well-being, continued good sleep health
Case 4: Emma	Regular exercise, active participation in support networks	Sustained energy levels, ongoing mental health support

🤩 THERE IS A SURPRISE FOR YOU 🤩

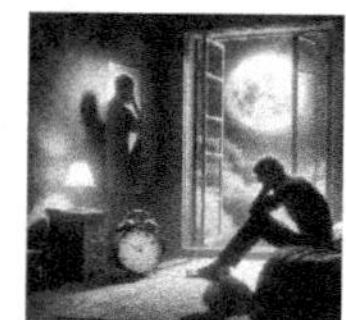

Scan Now for

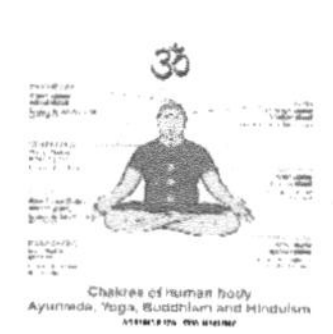

Double Bonus!!

What Will You Receive by Scanning Above?

- **An Easy and Comprehensive Guide** to provide the reader with in-depth and well-researched to address insomnia and sleep apnea.
- **Practical Tips, Techniques and Copy Strategies** that each one can apply in their daily lives, to enjoy a better life!!

A positive review is much appreciated. Thank you!!
https://www.amazon.com/review/create-review?&ASIN=B0CW19TGPG

Adrienne Fox

StayHealthy 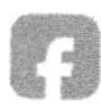 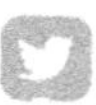 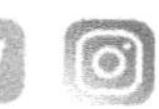 

misterbondwriter@gmail.com

www.ingramcontent.com/pod-product-compliance
Lightning Source LLC
Chambersburg PA
CBHW080853260726
48660CB00009B/3292